FROM STOLEN INTELLECT TO A GENIUS REVOLUTION

Awakening a Movement to Heal Generations

CATRINA GOODEN RAVENEL, BSW

Copyright © 2026 by Catrina Gooden Ravenel

Library of Congress Control Number:
2025922110

Paperback ISBN: 979-8-9944663-2-2
Hardback ISBN: 979-8-9944663-0-8
eBook ISBN: 979-8-9944663-1-5

Genre: 1. Iodine Deficiency. 2. IQ. 3. Literacy.
4. Global Nutrition. 5. Parenting. 6. Healing.
Printed in the United States of America

10 9 8 7 6 5 4 3 2 1
First Edition

No part of this book may be reproduced, stored in a retrieval system, transmitted, or distributed in any form or by any means—electronic, mechanical, photocopying, recording, scanning, or otherwise—without the prior written permission of the publisher, except for brief quotations used in reviews or scholarly works.

This book is published by **Minerallymade LLC**, a trademarked entity. Minerallymade® and Mineral Momma™ are trademarks of Minerallymade LLC.

The information contained in this book is for educational and informational purposes only. It is not intended as medical advice, diagnosis, or treatment. The author and publisher are not licensed medical professionals. Readers should consult qualified healthcare providers regarding any medical or health-related decisions.

The author has made every effort to ensure accuracy; however, no warranty is expressed or implied. The publisher and author assume no responsibility for errors, omissions, or outcomes resulting from the use of this information.

Printed in the United States of America.

Medical Disclaimer

The information presented in this book and through Minerallymade materials is for educational and informational purposes only. It is not intended as medical advice, diagnosis, or treatment.

Always consult with a qualified healthcare provider, physician, or registered dietitian before making any changes to your diet, supplement routine, or medical care plan—especially if you are pregnant, nursing, have a medical condition, or are taking prescription medication.

Statements regarding nutrients, minerals, or natural products are not evaluated by the U.S. Food and Drug Administration (FDA). These products and practices are not intended to diagnose, treat, cure, or prevent any disease.

Minerallymade LLC, its founder, affiliates, or partners assume no liability for any injury, loss, or damages arising from the use or misuse of the information provided herein. By engaging with this material, you acknowledge that you are responsible for your own health decisions.

TABLE OF CONTENTS

Special Dedications 7
About The Cover 9
Preface: The Awakening 11
The Stolen Intellect Series 13
Introduction: My Awakening 15
Prologue: The Opening Bell 19

SECTION 1: GENERATIONAL INTELLIGENCE. 21
Chapter 1: The Mind is a Terrible Thing to Waste 23
Chapter 2: A Walk Down Memory Lane 25
Chapter 3: The Secret Is in The Salt. 29
Chapter 4: The Blueprint for Civilization 34
Chapter 5: America's Iodine Solution 44
Chapter 6: 1948. 52
Chapter 7: Sabotaged Before Birth. 61
Chapter 8: Placenta to Prison Pipeline 72
Chapter 9: The Keepers of the Spoon 83
Chapter 10: Seaweed Soup – A Bowl of Genius. 90
Chapter 11: The Gift of a Well-Nourished Mind. 93
Chapter 12: The Soul of a Nation. 98
Chapter 13: The Call to Action. 104
Chapter 14: A Nation's Iodized-Salt Program 106
Chapter 15: The Case for Public Health Reparations 111

SECTION 2: GENERATIONAL HEALTH & LONGEVITY 117
Chapter 16: Bread – Once A Symbol of Life. 119
Chapter 17: Experiment on Rats, Not God's People 126

Chapter 18: Hesitate Before You Celebrate................................131

Chapter 19: Without Vision, the People Perish 135

Chapter 20: Sisters, Activate Your Power: Prevent Hearing Loss 144

Chapter 21: Nosebleeds – What the Web Won't Cure, Mother Nature Will 146

Chapter 22: Vitamin E is Not a Luxury – It's a Healer!.........................151

Chapter 23: There is No 'Us' Without Selenium 159

Chapter 24: A Power Pair: Iodine and Selenium 169

Chapter 25: Brilliant Forever 174

Chapter 26: Nourish your Destiny..181

Chapter 27: The Darkness We Inherited...185

Chapter 28: Iodine: The Forgotten First Aid 192

Chapter 29: Mothers Wit 195

Chapter 30: B.B.I.B.L.E...202

Chapter 31: The Prostate Protection Code......................................211

Chapter 32: Penis Painting 216

Chapter 33: A Note to Boy Moms 219

Chapter 34: Mother Nature's Pharmacy 225

Epilogue: The Genius Revolution & Healing Movement Begins..................236

Selected References & Further Reading 241

About the Author 243

Bonus Chapter: Stolen Intellect, Recovering the Missing Link to Generational health 245

Stolen Intellect I - Book Review...247

A Special Thanks to My Readers 248

We are Minerallymade-Not Diseased Made...249

Miyeok guk – A Korean Tradition...254

More Links 256

Review Time!..258

Bring the Message to Your Community 260

Speaking & Teaching Engagements..261

Index 266

SPECIAL DEDICATIONS

To Divine Intelligence
Thank You for the firmament—earth, air, sea, and sun—
they are not just science, but together they form the perfect
cosmic recipe for our intelligence, good health, and longevity.
This is our inheritance - our birthright - our truth.

Sisters
Keepers of the womb and the wisdom.
May every practice and program that protects you—
seaweed and salt, iodine and sunlight—
lift you as you bring healthy and genius souls into the world.

Brothers
Your leadership matters. Your wellness matters.
May you heal, rise, and reclaim the brilliance
that was always your birthright.

To our sons and daughters
You were made to rise brilliant and whole,
to lead with courage and serve with love,
to fulfill the divine purpose written inside you.

Ase

ABOUT THE COVER

An Homage to Family, Legacy, and the Rebirth of a People

This cover is inspired by the **African Renaissance Monument in Dakar, Senegal**—a towering testament to strength, unity, and rebirth. Though the artwork on this book is not an exact replica, it echoes the monument's **spirit**, its **posture**, and its **message**:

A family stands together. A people rise together.

My mother was the first to teach me the power of an image – for it speaks a thousand words!

She often reflected on how, across centuries, the most iconic religious depictions rarely showed a full family—Jesus alone, or Mary with the child, always fragmented.

She believed this absence was intentional, part of a deeper erasure meant to weaken the image of the family unit in the minds of colonized people.

Her insight stayed with me.

She taught me what it truly means when we say *pictures speak louder than words*. Images shape identity. And reclaiming our own visual language is part of how we heal.

But I must also honor my father—**the man whose presence shaped my courage**.

My father was not absent; he was firmly and actively in our home. A hardworking man, a veteran, a truck driver who traveled long roads to care for his family. Both Dad and Mom were activists and truth-seekers. They taught me to be a thinker and to be unafraid - to ask questions and uncover what others overlook.

Their steadiness formed the backbone of my strength, and together their love sharpened my mind. So, this cover reflects both: my mother's wisdom and my father's courage—my first models of unity.

And so, this image represents more than a monument.

It represents my parents,

my lineage,

our people,

and our return to wholeness.

To the people of Senegal, I offer my deepest respect.

May this homage be received not as appropriation, but as admiration—a heartfelt salute to a monument that awakened something ancient inside me. Your creation inspired a message that now lives through these pages.

The family on the cover stands for more than generational intelligence.

It stands for generational **dignity**.

It honors:

Family as foundation.
Community as keepers.
Mothers as the first physicians.
Fathers as protectors of legacy.
Children as the continuation of our brilliance.

This cover carries the vision my parents planted in me, and the vision I now return to the world:

A healed family becomes a healed nation.
A healed nation becomes a healed people.
And a healed people become unstoppable.

Artist-
Malcolm Turpin – digital artist and murals
Atlanta, Ga
malcolmturp@gmail.com

PREFACE

THE AWAKENING

*"When the ancestors whisper, the wise listen.
When the body breaks, the soul speaks."*

The cosmic recipe never changed.
It was written in the beginning—etched into earth, air, sea, and sun.
But our understanding of how these elements heal us, sustain us,
and protect us from disease…
was stolen, buried, and forgotten.
When these sacred elements vanished from our tables,
and when our bodies were flooded with toxic chemicals,
future generations became dimmer, weaker, more compromised.
What we call "disease" is often nothing more than
the absence of the ingredients we were designed to receive.
This book is a time capsule of *remembrance*.
We were meant to remember the cosmic recipe.
Remember the sea's minerals.
Remember the earth's foods.
Remember the air.
Remember the light.
Everything we need to heal—already given.
But what comes next is not just a health message.
It is a call across time—
a revolution of spirit and soil.
A summons to fight for the earth,
to guard our lands,
to cleanse our seas,

to heal our families,
and to pray for the end of all that brings us harm.
Now—
Gabriel's trumpet is sounding.
Not from distant mountains or ancient skies,
but in kitchens, in classrooms, in nations.
Do you hear it?
That…
is the Opening Bell.
The movement begins.

THE STOLEN INTELLECT SERIES

From Awakening → To Revolution

In my first book, *Stolen Intellect*, recovering the missing link to generational health, we exposed what was taken—the minerals, the elements, and the truth that shaped our brilliance.

We uncovered the quiet theft of health, potential, and generational power.

But revelation is only the beginning.

Once you know what was taken, you cannot remain silent. You cannot stay still.

This book marks the turning point.

From Stolen Intellect → to *A Genius Revolution* is the moment awakening becomes *action*, the moment remembering becomes *rebuilding*.

This is the blueprint for restoring our families, our children, our communities—and reclaiming the brilliance the world tried to steal.

Welcome to the movement.

INTRODUCTION

MY AWAKENING

*Every generation leaves clues about what it valued most —
its health, its children, its wisdom, and its food.*

**In the space between research and revelation,
the Universe began calling me.**

The more I listened, the clearer the answer became. I had come to this earth to help unlock human potential, and above all, to help us remember what we were never meant to forget.

I asked myself whether I was discovering my purpose—or if my purpose had discovered me. And as that question settled, something profound unfolded: every truth I had found pointed back to the same source.

The Four Cosmic Elements needed for life weren't symbols or lessons from childhood—they were the original instructions for human intelligence and survival.

Earth, air, sea, and sun are not just science and textbook lessons - they are the divine blueprint for nourishing the mind, sustaining the body, and restoring what has been stolen from us.

We were created to inherit the *full* recipe, born with the wisdom to use all four elements as they were designed- *together.* But the truth is this: some receive all four elements, but most do not.

Others grow up surviving with only three elements. Millions survive on two. And billions live with nothing but fragments of the original blueprint — the one meant to nourish intelligence, protect the body, and sustain life on this planet – the firmament.

How can the firmament be abundant, yet so many lack what it freely provides?

Here's my point. If you have all the ingredients to bake a cake using your grandmother's favorite recipe, you expect the outcome to be a perfect cake every time—and it is. But what happens when you miss just one ingredient? What if you miss two ingredients?

Well, the firmament is our perfect recipe.

So what happened?

Here is my message:

When a person is gifted with the fullness of the four elements, they carry within them the blueprint for genius, health, and longevity that can ripple through generations.

Miss one element

And the imbalance begins. A person may shine with intelligence yet wrestle with emotional storms or health problems that rise quietly and follow them through life.

Miss Two Elements

The consequences become more visible. People often experience unpredictable levels of cognition — shifting between moments of sharpness and periods of learning difficulty. Thyroid disorders, weak immunity, infertility, miscarriages, weight struggles, and slow development in children become common.

With Only One Element

A single element cannot hold the weight of human life. With only one, the body grows weary, the mind dims, and the spirit loses direction. Children grow up requiring wheelchairs and walkers, adults lose resilience, and the entire system begins to unravel. Nothing can flourish on one ingredient alone.

With Only Fragments

And when all that remains are fragments — scattered pieces of a design meant to be whole — we see it everywhere: unstable minds, fragile immunity, chronic illness, and generations losing their brilliance before it can bloom. Embryos miscarry. A fragmented foundation cannot support a thriving life. It can only produce struggle or not survive at all.

This is why supplementing to maintain perfect balance is critical! I know this reality intimately. Born in Detroit Michigan and growing up living in Inkster, Michigan—Where the Beautiful Great Lakes pull the minerals from the soil, where sunlight is scarce and the sea is nowhere near—my family lived with only two cosmic ingredients most of the time.

That deficiency shaped our lives. In the next generation, when my son was diagnosed with a learning disability, my spirit was shaken awake.

It was a spiritual slap—abrupt, painful, undeniable.

I thought I was following the Most High…

but I had been following the indoctrination of the *most low.*

As time passed, patterns revealed themselves everywhere: longevity for some, premature death for others; genius in one household, learning disabilities in the next.

When I was told my child might be born with profound learning challenges, my world shattered.

But that shock was also my awakening.

It jolted me out of a deep sleep and into a new reality.

Then, I saw my people were being led—but in the wrong direction.

And so, my divine assignment began. Clarity flooded in. I saw how mass manipulation and quiet deception had shaped our health for generations.

Insights poured in. People began telling me, *"I wish I'd known you before my best friend died,"* or *"before my sister was gone."* I feel the weight of their pain. Through it all, I learned one unshakable truth: **The cosmic recipe never changed!**

PROLOGUE

THE OPENING BELL

Sound the alarm — of the Genius Revolution.

It begins not in laboratories or lecture halls, but in kitchens, classrooms, and living rooms where minds are quietly starving.

It begins where mothers mix formula instead of minerals, where children are fed but not nourished, where brilliance lies asleep beneath layers of deficiency.

It begins where we remember: genius was never lost—only stolen.

Every page that follows is both an alarm and a remedy—an urgent call to recover the nutrients that build intelligence and restore the health our ancestors once protected.

These vitamins and minerals can help prevent blindness, support stroke recovery, strengthen immunity, reduce an enlarged heart, and even lower the risk of cancer.

No medical institution has the final say over our lives. So, when you find yourself desperately searching for ancient healing solutions, turn these pages.

This book is for women, for men, and for our children — because generational health, longevity, and genius are not miracles, but our natural birthright.

Here you will find the map back to the wisdom that once flowed from our ancestors' tables, guiding us toward stronger bodies, sharper minds, and a future filled with brilliance.

We are not waiting for policymakers or pharmaceuticals. We are waking up, one family at a time. This is not a diet trend. It's a return - A remembering.

Because when we feed the brain, we free the mind. When we nourish mothers, we heal nations. And when we restore the minerals of the earth to the people of the earth, brilliance, health, and strength rise again.

Welcome to the Genius Revolution!

And so, begins our shared mission: not just to awaken brilliance, but to restore it. The pages ahead will show you why this revolution matters, how it began, and how every family can join it—one meal, one mineral, one mind at a time.

SECTION 1

GENERATIONAL INTELLIGENCE

Chapters 1 - 15

CHAPTER 1

THE MIND IS A TERRIBLE THING TO WASTE

The Theft of Brilliance -Before the mind was dimmed, it was MAGNIFICENT. Before the numbers dropped, before the diagnoses multiplied, before classrooms turned into testing centers and creativity was replaced by compliance — there was BRILLIANCE.

Human intelligence was *never* meant to *decline*. The brain - designed by Creation to evolve, expand, restore and remember was hijacked by deficiency- a mineral one. The theft did not come with guns or chains this time — it came quietly, cunningly, through depleted soil, empty calories, but mostly by policies that favored profit over people.

Across generations, we have watched intelligence curve downward and illness curve upward. Each decade, more children are labeled, medicated, or misunderstood. Each year, more adults lose energy, clarity, and memory — calling it "aging" when it is really malnutrition in disguise.

This is not evolution.

It is erosion.

The land was stripped of minerals then policies stripped the mind. In the process, something sacred was stolen: our *cognitive inheritance*. The theft was slow, subtle, and systematic.

It began when governments ignored the mineral content of food and when they had the chance to replace it, they did not!

This book is a search party for what was lost.

Our *minds* are the most valuable thing we own. Not gold, copper or silver. Yet strangely too many children in America aren't getting nutrients to make the building blocks their brains need — not just to hit basic milestones, but to surpass them. Not just to be intelligent – but genius!

The Return of Genius

Recovery begins the moment we realize that food is not just fuel — it's code. Every bite sends a signal to the brain. But every mineral, every vitamin, every molecule whispers instructions to neurons - *grow, connect, communicate, remember.*

Neurons are specialized brain cells that *send and receive* information.

Your thoughts, memory, attention, mood, learning, and intelligence all depend on how well neurons:

- Grow
- Connect
- Communicate
- Maintain energy

This is the movement — not just nutritional, but generational. We are not chasing genius - we are restoring it. However, when a child's brain does not get the right minerals, school can't fix it.

These Headlines Speak Louder Than Any Protest

"Are we growing dumber? Americans' IQ scores drop in four of five measurements." (*John Anderer, March 22, 2023*)

1. "Illiteracy affects 18% of U.S. adults—57.4 million people. Most commonly impacting Black, Hispanic, and low-income individuals." (*Chloe Haderlie and Alyssa Clark, Fall 2017*)
2. "About 130 million adults in the U.S. have low literacy skills—more than half read below a sixth-grade level." (*Emily Schmidt, March 16, 2022*)
3. "Increase in developmental *disabilities* among children in the United States." (*CDC, Pediatrics Journal*)

This is not just a crisis of education. It is a crisis of **intellect, potential, and destiny.**

CHAPTER 2

A WALK DOWN MEMORY LANE

The Forgotten Origins of Iodine & Intelligence

1788 — Deep in the Alps

The year was 1788. Snow crowned the Alps like ancient white temples, and the mountain air carried echoes across the valleys of Switzerland. Travelers who journeyed through these isolated villages wrote of quiet tragedies hidden in plain sight.

Children walked with small, stunted bodies, their legs bowed like soft tiny trees starved of sunlight. Adults moved slowly, necks swollen with heavy goiters, eyes dulled not by age but by something deeper—something no one yet had language for.

In his travel guide, *Guide du Voyageur en Suisse*, Thomas Martyn described the "cretins" of the Valais. He did not know the word **iodine**. No one did. But he knew something was terribly wrong.

Imagine a mother in 1788 holding her infant. The child's cry is soft, the milestones delayed, the spark missing. She cannot name the problem. She cannot fix it. She simply endures it—generation after generation—passing down what she thinks is fate, when in truth, it was *a missing mineral the sea gives freely*.

What the travelers witnessed was not a curse nor was it destiny. It was **congenital iodine deficiency**, the most preventable cause of intellectual disability (*learning disabilities*) known to humanity.

Yet in the mountains, far from the ocean's gifts, this deficiency carved itself into family lines like an invisible inheritance of sorrow.

Within Just One Generation — The Mystery Begins to Break

Then, quietly, the world began to change.

1811 — A spark

A chemist studying burnt seaweed ash identifies a mysterious new substance. He calls it **iodine**.

He has no idea he has found the key to *unlocking human intelligence in entire nations.*

1820 — A breakthrough

In Geneva, Dr. Jean-François Coindet takes a bold risk. He gives iodine drops to patients with swollen necks.

To everyone's astonishment, the goiters shrink.

Mothers begin whispering through the community that a doctor has found *"the ocean in a bottle."*

1830s — A visionary in the Andes, South America

French chemist Boussingault studies entire villages in the mountains of South America and suggests something revolutionary:

"If the people lack iodine because they are far from the sea…then add iodine to the salt. Give iodine to everyone."

This was the first blueprint for the iodized salt programs that would one day protect *billions – humanity even.*

By the early 1900s —one of Europe's most affected countries—faced a national emergency.

Switzerland - From Crisis to Transformation

Teachers wrote letters describing classrooms full of children who could not keep up.

Farmers wrote that *entire families* struggled with learning delays.

Doctors reported that some villages had goiter rates above 80%.

The Swiss Government listened.

1922 — Switzerland steps into the future

Salt iodization begins.
Not as a trial.
Not as a trend.

But as a **commitment to protect every mother and every child**, regardless of where they lived or what they earned.

One generation on iodine, then another. And slowly, something miraculous happens:

- **Cretinism vanishes.**
- Children begin performing better in school.
- Entire regions experienced a rise in IQ—**10-15 points or more.**
- The country known for endemic goiter becomes the country known for *innovation, precision, and education.*

One mineral did that!
One decision changed a nation!
Because when a nation restores iodine, it restores its future.

Why This Story Still Echoes Today

The account that opens this chapter is nearly two hundred and forty years old, yet it mirrors the crisis still ongoing right now, today across a few nations that have not iodized their salt.

So here we are.

Children still struggling—not because they lack potential, but because they lack iodine.

Mothers still go through pregnancy without knowing their thyroid is starving.

Families still inherit learning difficulties that are **preventable**, not personal.

And that is why I wrote this book.

To sound the alarm!

To break the silence.

To reconnect families to the forgotten element that once reshaped the destiny of entire nations.

To spark a **Genius Revolution**—one that begins with remembering the sea, remembering the firmament and remembering that intelligence is not an accident...

It is nourished.

It is protected.

It is reclaimed.

It is our divine birthright!

Our stolen birthright......

Note:
- Congenital = present at birth
- It can develop **during pregnancy**
- It does **not** mean inherited or genetic (though it can be)

CHAPTER 2 BIBLIOGRAPHY

1. **Thomas Martyn's 1788 book**
   Martyn, Thomas. *Guide du Voyageur en Suisse*. 1788.
   (If you later locate a publisher or edition, we can update it.)
2. **WHO, Swiss Federal Office of Public Health, ICCIDD/IGN reports**
   World Health Organization; Swiss Federal Office of Public Health; and International Council for Control of Iodine Deficiency Disorders. *Reports on the Elimination of Endemic Cretinism and Iodine Deficiency through Salt Iodization*. Various years.
   (Chicago allows "Various years" when multiple reports spanning decades are used.)
3. **Big Think article (2020)**
   Big Think. "The Shocking, Forgotten History of Cretinism." *Big Think*, 2020. https://bigthink.com.
4. **Zimmermann iodine research (historical review)**
   Zimmermann, Michael B. "Iodine Deficiency and Thyroid Disorders: A Historical Perspective." *Public Health Nutrition*

CHAPTER 3

THE SECRET IS IN THE SALT

Country: Kazakhstan

A seventh grader teased his classmate - **"You're acting slow—are you iodine-deficient or something?"**

Harsh, yes—but revealing. It proved the national iodized-salt campaign in Kazakhstan was working. Children were beginning to associate iodine with intelligence.

A Nation That Refused to Wait

When Kazakhstan discovered its children were shorter than expected, that classrooms were underperforming, and that entire regions were showing clear signs of iodine deficiency, the nation did not spend decades debating policy.

They *acted*.

They **fortified household salt** with iodine.

They **launched a nationwide education campaign**.

UNICEF amplified the message.

USAID funded equipment upgrades and potassium iodate.

Salt producers modernized their factories.

Posters, pamphlets, mascots, cartoons, and school programs reached every home.

The message traveled so far and so fast that even students became advocates.

The Classroom That Changed Everything

One morning, a teacher—fully trained in the iodized-salt initiative—asked her students to bring salt from home.

The next day, every child placed their family's salt on their desk.

But the boy labeled "slow"…..

His family's salt was **plain**—not a trace of iodine. In that moment, the truth burst open. A wave of relief washed over his face.

He wasn't slow.

He wasn't broken.

He wasn't doomed.

He wasn't intellectually disabled; he was simply missing a mineral his brain needed to spark.

And because he was still in middle school and his brain was still developing, there was still time. Iodized salt transformed him—quickly, quietly, and powerfully.

A Movement Strengthened by Children

Across Kazakhstan, children urged their parents to buy iodized salt. Community groups made flyers. Schools reinforced the message. Families listened.

It wasn't a learning disability institution who recognized the boy's deficiency.

It wasn't the education system.

It wasn't a health professional.

It was:

- **The teacher** — trained to spot iodine deficiency.
- **The classmate** — who read a pamphlet and connected the dots.
- **The middle school students** — who refused to let their brilliance be stolen.

Iodine for the World — But not for Americans

U.S. taxpayer dollars—channeled through USAID and implemented by UNICEF—funded iodized-salt campaigns across Europe, Africa, Asia, and Eurasia.

Yet in the United States, iodized salt sits on the shelf labeled "iodine" —It's the public-health equivalent of installing smoke alarms in every home with no batteries.

Each year, millions of American workers contribute hard-earned dollars to organizations such as UNICEF USA to fund iodine-deficiency prevention programs overseas—while the United States itself maintains no mandatory iodized-salt policy to protect its own mothers, infants, and children.

Kazakhstan: So, Dr. Sharmanov, the National Health Ministry, Ms. Sivryukova and others <u>**devised**</u> a marketing campaign — much of it ***paid for by American taxpayers,*** *through money given to UNICEF by the United States Agency for International Development (USAID).*

The Quote above is an excerpt from the original article: In Raising the World's I.Q., the Secret's in the Salt - The New York Times

What a Seventh Grader Knew

The teasing seventh grader revealed truth millions still don't know:
Iodine shapes cognitive potential before a child ever steps into a classroom.

Iodine—born from the ocean, delivered as simple iodized salt—fuels the thyroid, the brain's developmental partner.

Yet, in America, we received empty, feel-good campaigns with no nutritional foundation, just this:

- "A mind is a terrible thing to waste."
- "Reading is fundamental."
- "Read to your baby."
- "Read for 20 minutes a day."

But without iodine to build the brain's neurons, it was already well understood reading campaigns would not work.

If a baby is iodine-deficient in the womb and remains iodine-deficient outside the womb, no amount of tutoring, phonics, bedtime stories and storytelling can restore what the thyroid and brain never received.

So, parents—confused and desperate—seek intervention:

- pediatricians, neurologists, ophthalmologists
- speech, occupational, and physical therapists
- specialists, tutors, endless testing
- special-needs schools and programs

They chase answers only to meet **shrugs**.

Meanwhile, medical, educational, and governmental systems expand their industries, businesses and wealth on the backs of generational deficiencies—never intending to fix the root cause.

Kazakhstan reports: 100% Universal Literacy

100% literacy means: Every person can read and write well enough to:

- learn
- work
- understand health information
- participate fully in society

No one left behind.

Sustained Iodine Sufficiency: Stable, year-after-year iodine intake that:

- prevents brain damage
- prevents learning disabilities
- protects IQ
- protects pregnancies
- strengthens national intelligence

This is generational genius made visible.

Why Literacy and Iodine Cannot Be Separated

Iodine **builds** *the brain.*
Literacy **uses** *the brain.*
Functional literacy: means a person can:

- read instructions
- understand medicine labels
- use maps and schedules
- fill out forms
- comprehend information well enough to make decisions

When everyone in society reaches this level, everything changes—health, economics, lifespan, problem-solving, innovation, democracy, and family stability.

Imagine a society where:

Every child's brain is nourished.
Every adult's mind is educated.
Every home is protected.

That is the promise of generational genius—vibrant health paired with deep learning across families. And it all begins with a mineral so small you can't see it…

The secret was added to the salt. But the ocean has always held iodine.

CHAPTER 3 BIBLIOGRAPHY

1. **Iodine Global Network global scorecard**
   Iodine Global Network. *Global Scorecard of Iodine Nutrition in 2021*. Ottawa: Iodine Global Network, 2021. https://www.ign.org.

2. **UNICEF MICS (household iodized salt data)**
   UNICEF. *Multiple Indicator Cluster Surveys (MICS): Household Use of Iodized Salt*. Various years. https://mics.unicef.org.

3. **USAID micronutrient fortification page**
   U.S. Agency for International Development (USAID). *Nutrition: Fortification and Other Micronutrient Interventions*. n.d. https://www.usaid.gov/what-we-do/global-health/nutrition.

4. **WHO/UNICEF/IGN manual on IDD elimination**
   World Health Organization, UNICEF, and Iodine Global Network. *Assessment of Iodine Deficiency Disorders and Monitoring Their Elimination: A Guide for Programme Managers*. 3rd ed. Geneva: World Health Organization, 2007. https://www.who.int/publications/i/item/9789241595827.

5. **Andersson, Karumbunathan & Zimmermann — global iodine status**
   Andersson, Maria, Vinod Karumbunathan, and Michael B. Zimmermann. "Global Iodine Status in 2011 and Trends." *Thyroid* 22, no. 5 (2012): 530–537. https://pubmed.ncbi.nlm.nih.gov.

6. **WHO/UNICEF case study in food fortification**
   Allen, Lindsay, Brigitte de Benoist, Omar Dary, and Richard Hurrell, eds. "Case Study: Universal Salt Iodisation." In *Food Fortification in a Globalized World*. Oxford: Oxford University Press.

7. **New York Times article**
   McNeil, Donald G. Jr. "In Raising the World's I.Q., the Secret's in the Salt." *The New York Times*, December 16, 2006. https://www.nytimes.com.

8. **UNCF classic slogan**
   United Negro College Fund (UNCF). *A Mind Is a Terrible Thing to Waste*. Advertising campaign slogan, introduced 1972. United States.

CHAPTER 4

THE BLUEPRINT FOR CIVILIZATION

The Blueprint for a sound and intelligent civilization begins with minerals first and everything else second. Across the world, health leaders championed one of the most powerful public-health programs ever created on earth - **Universal Salt Iodization (USI)**.

Its purpose was simple but profound — protect women of childbearing age, pregnant mothers, breastfeeding mothers, and young children. These groups hold the key to breaking intergenerational iodine deficiency and building an intelligent nation.

It is the quiet force behind *global brainpower* — stretching across Asia, Africa, Europe, Canada, Mexico, and South America — and still, much of humanity has no idea that behind their intelligence such a program exists.

I travel. I meet brilliant people — professionals, parents, leaders, international college students, thinkers and school principals. Yet when I ask about the global iodized-salt program that boosts IQ, literacy, generational intelligence and a strong nation, they all say the same words: **"I've never heard of it."**

The greatest threat to humanity's most successful public-health program was never opposition—it was omission. A victory so complete it was removed from education, stripped from memory, and left undefended. What is not taught cannot be guarded. What is not guarded will be lost. And what is lost will have to be relearned—at the cost of human potential.

1. **Successful prevention programs are often erased by their own success**
   When crises disappear (goiter, cretinism, widespread cognitive impairment), people forget *why* they disappeared.
2. **Education is the immune system of policy**

If students are never taught about iodization, fortification, or micronutrient defense:

- They won't defend it as adults
- They won't fund it
- They won't update or modernize it

3. **Silence is not neutral—it is destabilizing**
Programs that rely on memory instead of education eventually collapse.

This is not opinion. This is how collective intelligence is quietly eroded:

- **Iodine programs weakened in the United States**
- **Selenium knowledge vanished from medical training**
- **Prenatal nutrition became fragmented and commercialized**

Bottom line: when memory is stripped away, people stop remembering.
If students are never nourished, they cannot recall.
The aging population forgets what was never reinforced.
This is why **every person must know the Cosmic Recipe for Intelligence—** because what is not remembered cannot be protected!

The World's Promise: Protect Women, Protect the Babies, Protect the Future

The purpose of the global iodized salt program was clear:

- Nourish the thyroid of every mother and daughter.
- Support healthy pregnancies and healthy births.
- Strengthen intelligence for every generation.

How could mothers protect their families if they never knew about a program designed for them? How could fathers guard their homes when iodine - the first line of defense was hidden from them?

What Fathers Were Never Told

Do fathers know that iodine deficiency is the world's leading cause of preventable intellectual disability? Did anyone inform them the mineral iodine determines their child's:

- IQ
- language development
- attention span
- memory
- emotional stability (*the capacity to regulate emotions, tolerate stress, feel emotions without losing control, and to return to calm after challenges*).

So, fathers were left unarmed. Left watching their wives struggle with thyroid problems, miscarriages, fatigue, and hormonal confusion — not because they failed, but because their nation failed to educate them.
A father who knows is a father who defends.
A father informed becomes a keeper of brainpower, destiny, and generations.
Minerals Shape Nations!

IQ Is Nutritional Before It Is Educational

Many of the people who live in countries transformed by iodine — where literacy blooms and brilliance rises — often credit their schools, curriculum, or discipline. But rarely the mineral that made their intellect possible.

The Biological Connection Between Minerals and Genius

Across the world, we often describe entire nations with a single stroke:
"Ethiopians are intelligent."
"The Chinese are disciplined and brilliant."
"Island populations are sharp and long-lived."
These reputations do not emerge from thin air or come from DNA alone. They come from **biology**— from the *consistent presence* of the minerals that build and protect the human brain. And they form when consistent systems—education, nourishment, cultural expectation, and public policy—shape human potential over time.
A nation's genius does not begin in the university.
It begins **in the womb**.

Individual Genius vs. National Genius

In the United States, we tend to identify intelligence at the **individual level**. We say *he* is intelligent or *she* is gifted.

We marvel when:

- a three-year-old reads early, or
- a four-year-old can name all the presidents.

These children are celebrated as exceptions.

But in many parts of the world, **genius is not rare—it is common** because the biological foundations are protected across generations.

Minerals Build Minds That Build Nations

Iodine builds the brain.
Selenium protects it.
Iron fuels it.
Omega-3s wire it.

Note: *Cod Liver Oil contains omega 3s. There is no vegetarian cod liver oil. What exists instead is algae oil—the original marine source of omega-3s—which can replace DHA and EPA, but not the fat-soluble vitamins that only animal livers provide.*

What does "fat-soluble" mean?

Fat-soluble nutrients are vitamins and compounds that:

- **Dissolve in fat (not water)**
- **Must be eaten with fat to be absorbed**
- **Are stored in the body** (liver, brain, fatty tissues)
- **Build and protect structures** rather than acting quickly and leaving

Think of fat-soluble nutrients as **long-term builders and guardians** of the body.

The fat-soluble vitamins

Vitamin A

- Vision (retina, night vision)
- Brain development

- Immune defense
- Epithelial tissue (eyes, lungs, gut)

Found in: cod liver oil (retinol), red palm oil (carotenoids)

Vitamin D

- Brain signaling
- Immune regulation
- Bone & nerve development
- Gene expression (turns genes on/off)

Found in: cod liver oil, sunlight, some animal fats

Vitamin E

- Protects nerves and brain cells
- Prevents fat oxidation
- Supports fertility and circulation

Found in: red palm oil (especially tocotrienols), seeds, nuts

Vitamin K

- Blood clotting
- Bone strength
- Works with vitamin D to place calcium correctly

Found in: leafy greens (K1), fermented foods & animal fats (K2)

Why fat-soluble nutrients are so powerful

Unlike water-soluble vitamins (*like vitamin C or B-complex*), fat-soluble nutrients:

- Accumulate overtime
- Cross the blood–brain barrier
- Shape development in the womb
- Protect future generations

This is why deficiencies show up as:

- Vision problems
- Learning disabilities
- Immune weakness
- Fertility and pregnancy complications

A, D, E, and K ride in on fat. Without fat, they don't get in.
This is a *quiet failure point* in modern supplementation:

- People "take vitamin D"
- Blood levels stay low
- Doctors increase the dose
- The real problem was **delivery**, not deficiency

The **Cosmic Recipe** always paired fat-soluble nutrients with fat—modern pills often separate what nature never did.

This is why entire populations can be described as:

- *intellectually strong*
- *innovative*
- *disciplined*
- *resilient*
- *long-lived*

Not because of superiority—but because of **nutritional continuity**.

Minerals Build National Brilliance

- iodine
- selenium
- iron
- vitamin A
- omega-3 fats (DHA, EPA, ALA)
- seaweed and seafood
- clean soil

- sunshine
- ancestral food traditions

Where these remain intact, brilliance remains intact. Where these are stolen or forgotten, intelligence declines. These nutrients shape:

- thyroid hormone (the engine of brainpower)
- heart strength (oxygen for the brain)
- nervous system speed and clarity
- emotional stability
- creativity and problem-solving capacity

This is why coastal nations, volcanic-soil nations, and traditional cultures consistently display strong collective intellect due to mineral continuity.

Ethiopia: Volcanic Soil, Mineral-Rich Diets — and a Strong Iodized Salt Program

Ethiopia's volcanic soil is naturally rich in minerals that nourish both body and mind. But Ethiopia also did something some nations failed to do: **they implemented a universal iodized-salt program** to protect the brains of mothers, infants, and future generations.

Ethiopia's Iodized-Salt Journey: A Quiet Victory for National Intelligence

Ethiopia was not late to recognize the importance of iodine. The nation first introduced a salt-iodization effort in the **late 1980s**, aiming to prevent widespread learning disabilities and thyroid disorders caused by iodine deficiency.

However, regional shifts—especially the separation of Eritrea and disruptions in salt production in the late 1990s and early 2000s—caused coverage to collapse. Large populations once again faced preventable iodine deficiency. Realizing the danger, Ethiopia corrected course.

On **March 25, 2011**, the government passed a **mandatory iodized-salt law**, banning the sale of non-iodized salt for human consumption. This single policy restored the nation's shield of protection.

And the results were swift: by **2016**, nearly **90% of Ethiopian households** had access to iodized salt.

Today, Ethiopia stands among the nations that actively protect the brains of their mothers, babies, and future generations—demonstrating what happens when a country sees iodine not as optional, but as essential.

And the pattern became clear - The farther from the ocean, the more the human brain suffers.

China's Iodine Shield: Protecting a Billion Minds

China's iodine story is not one of failure—it is one of **responsibility at scale**.

By the late twentieth century, China faced a reality few nations have ever confronted: iodine deficiency disorders affected **hundreds of millions of people** across vast inland and mountainous regions. In some provinces, generations of children were born with preventable learning disabilities, growth impairment, and thyroid disease—not from neglect, but from geography.

Far from the sea, iodine had simply disappeared from daily life.

China did not deny the problem.

Public-health surveys revealed what science already knew: iodine deficiency was quietly reducing national intelligence, child by child, womb by womb. And unlike conditions that require decades of medical treatment, iodine deficiency had a known, *affordable, and proven solution.*

So, China acted.

A National Commitment to Intelligence

In 1995, China implemented **Universal Salt Iodization**, making iodized salt the standard for human consumption across the country. This was not framed as medicine or charity—it was framed as **protection**.

Salt production was *regulated*.

Iodine levels were *standardized*.

Monitoring systems were established.

Education followed policy.

The goal was clear: **no child's brain should be sacrificed to geography**.

The Quiet Results

Within years, the change was unmistakable.

Goiter rates in school-aged children fell sharply.

Severe iodine-deficiency disorders nearly disappeared.

Entire regions once labeled "endemic" recovered.

Tens of millions of children were spared irreversible brain damage.

Public-health experts later described China's iodized-salt program as **one of the largest cognitive-protection efforts in human history**—not because it was dramatic, but because it was effective.

No slogans.

No fanfare.

Just salt—restored.

What China Understood

China recognized a truth many nations still resist:

Intelligence is not merely inherited or taught.

It is **nourished**.

By treating iodine as a foundational nutrient—rather than an optional supplement—China acknowledged its duty not only to the present generation, but to the unborn.

This was not about raising test scores.

It was about **protecting human potential before it could be lost**.

A Lesson for the World

China's experience confirms what Switzerland first observed, what Kazakhstan taught its children, and what Ethiopia courageously restored:

When iodine returns to the table, intelligence returns to the nation.

Different cultures.

Different systems.

Same mineral.

Same result.

China's iodized-salt program stands as proof that safeguarding intelligence is not ideological—it is **biological**. And when a nation chooses prevention over diagnosis, the benefits ripple quietly across generations.

Some nations build monuments of stone. Others build monuments of policy. China chose salt—and protected a *billion minds* without saying a word.

CHAPTER 4 BIBLIOGRAPHY

1. **WHO/UNICEF Guidance on Iodine Supplementation (2023)** World Health Organization and UNICEF. *Iodine Supplementation in Pregnant and Lactating Women: Guidance Summary*. Geneva: World Health Organization, 2023.

2. **UNICEF Global Iodine Coverage Data** UNICEF. *Iodine: Global Coverage and Equity of Iodized Salt*. UNICEF Data, c. 2020. https://data.unicef.org.

3. **Zimmermann & Andersson — Global iodized salt coverage**
Zimmermann, Michael B., and Maria Andersson. "Coverage of Iodized Salt Programs and Iodine Status in 2020." *European Journal of Endocrinology* (review and data synthesis; year varies).

4. **Qian et al. Meta-analysis on iodine & intelligence** Qian, Meiyun, Yuji Kawashima, Annette S. A. Z. Ruhija, Basil Hetzel, et al. "The Effects of Iodine on Intelligence in Children: A Meta-Analysis." *American Journal of Clinical Nutrition* 81, no. 1 (2005): 220–225.

5. **Bougma et al. — Iodine & early childhood mental development** Bougma, Kouanda, N. Aboudou, J. Christiansen, and M. Zimmermann. "Iodine and Mental Development of Children 5 Years Old and Under." *Nutrients* 5, no. 4 (2013): 1384–1416.

6. **Bath et al. — Low iodine status in UK pregnancy & child cognition** Bath, Sarah C., Margaret P. Rayman, Jane L. Steer, et al. "Low Iodine Status in UK Pregnant Women and Cognitive Outcomes in Their Children." *The Lancet* 382 (2013): 331–337.

7. **Leung, Pearce & Braverman — History of U.S. iodine fortification** Leung, Angela M., Elizabeth N. Pearce, and Lewis E. Braverman. "History of U.S. Iodine Fortification and Supplementation." *Thyroid* 22, no. 10 (2012): 1029–1036.

8. **Markel — "A Grain of Salt"** Markel, Howard. "A Grain of Salt." *The Milbank Quarterly* 92, no. 1 (2014): 123–149.

9. **Sun D et al.** *Eliminating Iodine Deficiency in China: Achievements and Challenges*, showing the national program's strategy and outcomes.

CHAPTER 5

AMERICA'S IODINE SOLUTION

"The Goiter Belt was not a failure of parenting or education.
It was a failure of minerals."

The Great Lakes Region Before 1924: An Iodine-Deficiency Crisis

Before 1924, iodine deficiency quietly compromised the intelligence, growth, and physical development of millions living in the Great Lakes region. Iodized salt changed that—almost overnight.

Where this occurred

The iodine-deficient zone stretched across:

- The **Great Lakes states** (Michigan, Ohio, Indiana, Illinois, Wisconsin)
- The **Upper Midwest**
- Inland regions far from the ocean
- Places where glaciers (ice) long ago scraped the land, washing away iodine from the soil.

Glaciation refers to long periods in Earth's history—**Ice Ages**—when massive sheets of ice (glaciers) covered large parts of the land.
These glaciers were:

- *Miles thick*
- *Slow-moving*
- *As powerful as bulldozers*

As they moved, they **scraped, crushed, and stripped** the land beneath them.

Repeated glaciation had stripped iodine from the soil. Food grown there contained **very little iodine**, and people had **no supplementation**. Geographically, they were far from the ocean.

Low Iodine Deficiency Affected Different Groups

Children

Children were the **most visibly affected**.

Common outcomes included:

- **Goiter** (enlarged thyroid)
- Delayed growth
- Poor concentration and memory
- Learning difficulties
- Speech and hearing problems
- Increased fatigue
- *Higher rates of special education needs* (though not named as such then)

In severe cases:

- **Cretinism** (intellectual disability, motor impairment)
- Poor coordination and delayed walking
- Short stature
- Skeletal abnormalities

Common Skeletal Abnormalities

Bone Shape & Growth

- **Rickets** – soft, weak bones in children due to vitamin D deficiency
- **Bowed legs** – legs curve outward or inward from weak bones
- **Short stature** – bones do not grow to expected height
- **Delayed bone growth** – bones mature more slowly than normal

Spine & Posture

- **Scoliosis** – sideways curve of the spine
- **Kyphosis** – rounded upper back ("hunchback")
- **Lordosis** – exaggerated inward curve of the lower back

Skull & Face

- **Abnormal skull shape** – skull does not grow evenly
- **Delayed closure of soft spots (fontanelles)**
- **Narrow jaw or crowded teeth** – jaw does not widen properly

Joints & Movement

- **Joint stiffness** – reduced range of motion
- **Poor alignment of joints** – knees, hips, or ankles misaligned
- **Delayed walking** – difficulty learning to stand or walk on time

Congenital (Present at Birth)

- **Limb length differences** – one arm or leg shorter
- **Extra or missing bones**
- **Malformed hands or feet**

Nutrition-Related Skeletal Abnormalities

- **Rickets** (vitamin D & calcium deficiency)
- **Weak or brittle bones** (mineral deficiency)
- **Poor spinal support** (iodine, selenium, vitamin D interplay)
- **Delayed motor development** (brain–bone signaling issues)

Teachers and physicians regularly reported:

"Children who could not keep up, not because they were lazy, but because they were slow to process."

Women (especially pregnant women)

Women suffered *profoundly*—often invisibly.
Common effects:

- Goiter (especially during pregnancy)
- Miscarriages and stillbirths
- Difficult labor
- Postpartum exhaustion
- Thyroid failure *later in life*

Most critically:

- Iodine-deficient mothers gave birth to iodine-deficient babies
- This compromised brain development *in the womb*
- Damage was **often permanent**

This is why iodine is now recognized as essential for pregnancy.

Men

Men were also affected, though less often diagnosed.
Symptoms included:

- Goiter
- Low energy and endurance
- Reduced work capacity
- Slowed thinking
- Depression and apathy

In industrial regions (factories, farms, railroads), this translated to:

- Lower productivity
- Higher injury rates
- Poor recovery from illness

Late 1800s – The Silent Pattern Emerges

- Physicians notice unusually high rates of **goiter** in inland regions of the United States.
- The **Great Lakes and Upper Midwest** stand out.
- Coastal populations show **far fewer thyroid problems**.
- Cause not yet fully named, but geography is suspected.

1890–1905 – The "Goiter Belt" Is Identified

- Medical journals begin referring to a broad inland zone as the **"Goiter Belt."**
- This includes Michigan, Ohio, Indiana, Illinois, Wisconsin, and surrounding states.
- Food grown locally lacks iodine.

1906–1915 – Children Reveal the Crisis

School health inspections show:

- **30–65% of children** in some towns have enlarged thyroids
- Teenage girls are especially affected (largely due to *breasts growing and menstrual cycle flowing*)

Teachers report:

- Poor concentration
- Slowed learning
- Fatigue

These children are often mislabeled as "slow" or "weak."

1916–1920 – Pregnancy and Generational Impact Recognized

Doctors observe:

- High goiter rates in pregnant women
- Increased miscarriages and stillbirths
- Babies born with developmental delays

Researchers connect **maternal iodine deficiency** to:

- Impaired brain development in the womb
- Permanent cognitive and motor damage in severe cases

Parallels drawn to **Alpine cretinism** in Europe.

1917–1922 – Iodine as the Solution

European studies confirm:

- Iodine supplementation prevents goiter
- Seaweed and seafood are protective

U.S. researchers conduct trials using iodine drops and iodine-rich foods.

Results:

- Goiters shrink
- Energy improves
- Children function better in school

World War I (1917–1918): When Iodine Deficiency Reached the Draft Office

1917 – America Enters World War I

As the United States mobilized for war, millions of young men reported for military examinations. What doctors and recruiters found was alarming.

Across the Great Lakes region and other inland areas:

- **Goiters were widespread**
- Many men showed signs of **thyroid dysfunction**
- Fatigue, weakness, and slowed reflexes were common
- Some recruits were deemed **unfit for service**

Goiter was not cosmetic—it was a sign of **impaired thyroid function**, which affects:

- Endurance
- Muscle strength
- Heart rate
- Cognitive sharpness
- *Stress tolerance*

All critical for soldiers.

Recruitment Struggles

Military physicians reported:

- High rejection rates in iodine-poor regions
- Disproportionately affected inland states
- ***Better physical readiness among men from coastal areas***

The pattern mirrored civilian data:
Where iodine was scarce, bodies struggled.
This was no longer just an education problem—it was a defense issue too.

A National Wake-Up Call

World War I forced the U.S. government and medical community to confront an uncomfortable truth:

- A mineral deficiency was weakening the population
- The problem began **before adulthood**
- It affected men, women, and children alike
- Education and patriotism could not override biology

Healthy armies require **nourished bodies**.

Post-War Medical Consensus (1919–1923)

After the war:

- Military medical data reinforced civilian findings
- Physicians emphasized prevention, not treatment
- Maternal and childhood nutrition gained urgency
- Iodine deficiency was recognized as **avoidable**

1924 – The Turning Point

- **Iodized salt is introduced in the United States.**
- **Michigan becomes the pilot state**, chosen because of extreme goiter prevalence.
- Salt companies cooperate *voluntarily*.
- Public-health messaging focuses on **prevention**, especially for children and mothers.

1925–1930 – A Public Health Miracle

- Goiter rates drop **dramatically** within just a few years.
- New cases of cretinism nearly disappear.

- Children grow *taller, stronger, and more alert.*
- One of the **fastest and most successful nutrition interventions in U.S. history.**

1 generation (18 years) later.....

CHAPTER 6

1948

When lawmakers voted down mandatory iodized salt in *1948*, they didn't merely deny a micronutrient — they sentenced a nation to illiteracy, physical disability, slow decline, mass incarceration, premature death and chaos!

That vote was a silent theft: of children's learning, of mothers' strength, of grandparents' long memory and longevity. For decades we have paid with severe to moderate intellectual impairment. This was a choice with a human cost in America - this was not an accident!

The United States had everything—science, funding, proof, and global guidance. The door to protection stood wide open. Yet from 1948 to present, this nation moved through twenty presidential elections and fifteen presidents and chose to look the other way.

Seventy-eight years later; fifteen (15) presidents later, and not one of them in office delivered the protection that could have saved multiple generations.

When harm persists this long in the presence of knowledge, it is no longer ignorance. It is policy. The result is not an accident. It is catastrophic, manufactured, and generational.

The American Contrast: A Reversal of Genius

America's decline did not happen because:

- mothers stopped caring
- fathers stopped leading
- teachers stopped teaching
- children stopped trying

The decline began when **minerals disappeared**:

- iodine vanished from the table
- selenium declined in the soil
- iron deficiency became common
- ultra-processed food replaced nourishment
- bromate replaced iodine in the bread
- the womb was left unprotected

A population cannot think, learn, innovate, or excel without the minerals that make intelligence possible! People did not become less worthy. They became less nourished.

Intelligence and physical ability are built by the same foundation

Iodine, selenium, vitamin D, and iron—the supreme gifts of the sea, sun, air, and earth—do more than shape how the mind works; they guide how the brain directs the body to form, grow, and thrive.

The Architect Behind Intelligence and Health

Each neuron has three main parts:

1. **Cell body** – keeps the neuron alive
2. **Axon** – sends messages outward
3. **Dendrites** – receive messages from other neurons

Intelligence is not about how many neurons you have alone—it's about how well they connect, collaborate and communicate.

Dendrites: Where Intelligence Is Built

Dendrites look like tiny tree branches extending from neurons.
Their role:

- Receive incoming signals
- Form connections (synapses) with other neurons
- Create neural networks

The more healthy, complex, and well-branched dendrites you have, the more:

- Information you can process
- Memories you can store
- Patterns you can recognize
- Reasoning you can perform

Dendritic growth = learning capacity

This is why early life nutrition is so critical.

Iodine: The Architect Behind Neural Growth

Iodine and selenium does not act directly on neurons—it works through the thyroid hormones (T3 and T4) that guide brain development.

Thyroid hormones control

- Neuron migration (where neurons settle in the brain)
- Dendritic branching and complexity
- Synapse formation
- Myelination (speed of signal transmission)
- Brain energy metabolism

Growing up away from the sea in the United States, that foundation was incomplete

- Neurons form incorrectly
- Dendrites are shorter and fewer
- Neural networks are sparse
- Learning capacity is reduced

When iodine is missing—especially during pregnancy

- Fewer dendrites form
- Synapses are weaker
- Brain regions do not mature on schedule
- IQ can be reduced by 10–15 points or more
- Attention, memory, and language suffer

Intelligence Is a Network, Not a Number

Intelligence emerges from:

- Dense dendritic trees
- Strong synaptic connections
- Efficient communication
- Adequate energy supply

Iodine is foundational because it **sets the blueprint** for all of this.
If iodine is missing early:

- No amount of schooling can fully correct it.
- Education builds on what biology allows.
- When these minerals are missing during development, both learning and movement can suffer.

How This Connects to Physical Disability

Your brain doesn't just help you think—it also helps your body **move, grow, and stay strong**.
Neurons send messages from the brain to the muscles.
These messages tell your body how to:

- Walk
- Run
- Hold things
- Keep balance
- Coordinate movements

The better the brain cells are built, the better these messages travel.

Why Iodine Matters for the Body

Iodine helps the brain and nervous system grow **before a baby is born** and during early childhood.
Iodine helps:

- Brain cells connect properly

- Messages travel quickly and clearly
- Muscles get the right signals
- Bones and muscles grow on time

Like the telephone game, where whispers lose their truth as they travel, biological messages can fade across generations. *Iodine preserves the signal.*

What Happens When Iodine Is Missing

If iodine is missing during pregnancy or early life:

- Messages to the muscles can be slow or mixed up
- Balance and coordination may be harder
- Muscle control may be weak

This can lead to **physical challenges**, such as:

- Trouble walking or running
- Poor coordination
- Weak muscles
- Delayed growth
- Difficulty with fine motor skills (like writing)

Brain and Body Work Together

The brain is like the **control center**, and the body is like the **machine**. If the control center doesn't send clear messages, the machine can't work properly.

In Short:

Deliberate iodine deficiency is a crime against humanity because it:

- **Steals intelligence before birth**, permanently lowering a population's cognitive potential.
- **Creates preventable learning disabilities**, mislabeling children as "slow," "special needs," or "behavioral problems" when they are nutritionally injured.
- **Shrinks generational capacity**, so each generation starts life with less than the one before it.

- **Weakens memory, reasoning, and judgment**, eroding a society's ability to think critically, innovate, and self-govern.
- **Increases dependence**, producing populations more vulnerable to control, misinformation, and exploitation.
- **Distorts education systems**, forcing schools to manage damage rather than cultivate brilliance.
- **Drives poverty across generations**, as impaired cognition limits opportunity, productivity, and economic mobility.
- **Overloads healthcare systems**, replacing prevention with lifelong treatment, disability services, and pharmaceuticals.
- **Breaks families**, as parents blame themselves or their children for outcomes rooted in policy failure.
- **Silences genius**, burying inventors, leaders, artists, and thinkers before they ever emerge.
- **Turns a nutrient deficiency into a social hierarchy**, where access to intelligence becomes accidental instead of protected.
- **Normalizes preventable harm**, teaching nations to accept decline as fate rather than policy choice.
- **Erases accountability**, allowing institutions to call the damage "genetic," "random," or "inevitable."
- **Undermines national security**, because a nation that cannot think clearly cannot protect itself.
- **Commits violence strategically**, without obvious bloodshed, but wounding generations of their intelligence and sound minds *quietly, strategically, legally, and at scale.*
- **Do No Harm – It's too late!**

The Blueprint of Civilization: Minerals First, Everything Else Second

Civilizations rise and fall not only because of armies or governing systems, but because of the micronutrients available to:

- mothers
- fathers
- babies
- the womb
- the soil

Minerals shape bodies.
Minerals shape minds.
Minds shape nations.
Nations shape history.
This is the unspoken truth behind:

- intelligence
- creativity
- innovation
- emotional stability
- national destiny

In America - The Atrocities Since 1948

More than 150 million Americans struggle to read — that's more people than the entire population of Japan. Imagine the vulnerability of a nation where half its citizens cannot read beyond a fifth-grade level. What happens when millions cannot fully comprehend the policies, contracts, warnings, or systems that govern their lives?

- The nation becomes exposed.
- It becomes unstable.
- It becomes easy to steer, mislead, and control.
- This is what happens when literacy collapses: a people lose their power, and a country loses its direction.

Reclaiming What Was Always Ours

We have not merely fallen behind—we have been quietly undone. Seventy-eight years have passed while the rest of the world rose up to defend the minds of their children, and America did not follow.

We turned away from a mineral that governs thought, memory, speech, and life itself, and in doing so, we reversed time. It is as if this nation has been pushed back to 1788—before the science, before the safeguards, before we understood that when iodine is missing, intelligence dims, voices are delayed, and destinies are quietly rerouted.

This is not a minor deficiency; it is a generational theft unfolding in silence. In classrooms where children struggle to speak, in wombs left unprotected, and in homes where no one was ever told what was missing, the cost has been immeasurable.

When a nation neglects the nourishment of the brain, it does not simply lose health—it forfeits wisdom, clarity, and its future.

So, I write first to Black people in America who have never lacked intelligence. What was disrupted was access to the biological protections that allow intelligence to fully express itself across generations.

The goal is not to prove that Black people are intelligent—we always have been.

The goal is for **America as a nation** to once again protect the biological foundations of genius, so intelligence is no longer rare, fragile, or unevenly distributed. When minerals are restored, intelligence becomes normal—and **genius becomes collective rather than exceptional**.

Brighter Futures for Others

<u>Brighter futures: Protecting early brain development through salt iodization - The UNICEF-GAIN Partnership Project - World | Relief Web</u>

"The nutrients a child receives in the earliest years of life influence their brain development for life and can make or break their chance of a prosperous future," said United Nations International Children's Emergency Fund -UNICEF Senior Nutrition Adviser Roland Kupka. "By protecting and supporting children's development in early life, we are able to achieve **immense results** for children *throughout their lifespan.*"

CLOSING TRUTH

Salt iodization is both cost effective and economically beneficial at only US $0.02–0.05 per child annually. **That's 2 to 5 cents per year per person!** Every dollar spent on salt iodization is estimated to return USD $30 through increased future cognitive ability.

A bright future depends on more than dreams, and determination depends on a brain that was given the tools to grow.

1922 – Dr. David Cowie, a pediatrician and chair of the Michigan Medical Society, proposed that the U.S. adopt salt iodization to eliminate goiter.

1924 – Iodized salt was introduced in Michigan. Morton Salt rolled out iodized salt nationally later that year.

1926 – Dr. Charles Hartsock, a thyroid surgeon, criticized iodized salt after observing cases of hyperthyroidism.

1934 – Those cases subsided. In fact, thyroid surgeries in Michigan hospitals dropped by **60%** after salt iodization. (*Less caseloads = less surgeries*)

1948 – The U.S. Endemic Goiter Committee proposed mandatory iodized salt for all states. The bill failed!

1951 – A Michigan survey found goiter rates had plummeted from 38.6% in 1924 to just 1.4%. Proof that iodized salt worked.

1975 – Congress enacted the *Education for All Handicapped Children Act (EHA)*—later renamed (Individual's Disability Education Act (IDEA) in 1990. These laws attempted to manage the fallout of widespread learning disabilities instead of preventing them.

2020 – According to the NIH, *124 countries* had mandatory iodized salt legislation. The U.S. was not one of them. Instead, it remained "voluntary"—a polite word that hides a brutal truth – a nation moving forward –without iodine.

CHAPTER 7

SABOTAGED BEFORE BIRTH

"Darkness covered the earth, but gross darkness covered the people" — and in the United States, that darkness took the shape of iodine deficiency, reshaped destinies, toxic and engineered foods, and whole generations living *without* the nutrients that keep the brain lit.

This wasn't a metaphor. It was a mineral crisis dressed up as normal life. A darkness that crept into our homes, our schools, our hospitals, and our communities.

Iodine is a micronutrient the body *cannot* make—and *nothing else* can replace its role in human development. As Velasco, Bath, and Rayman remind us - **iodine is *"an essential micronutrient"* during the first 1,000 days of life,** *when the foundations of thyroid health, brain wiring, and lifelong intelligence are laid* (Velasco, Bath & Rayman, 2018).

1000 Days – Starts from Conception to a Child's Second Birthday

The first 1,000 days are not just a developmental window—they are a biological contract. When the nutrients required to build life are missing, the body adapts. The cost of that adaptation is often paid by mothers first, and children next.

It is often around age two that parents begin to notice something is not right— delays in speech, vision, movement, or the need for early intervention services such as physical, occupational, or speech therapy.

During those earlier weeks of conception, I think of my cousin Rochelle who lives in Detroit. She was pregnant six times. In the first four pregnancies, each time the baby died in the womb. Calling it "miscarriage" makes Rochelle — and so many other women — believe it was something they did wrong, rather than something that was done to them. They were victims of a recurring tragedy, one whose outcome was already defined more than 78 years ago.

Eventually, Rochelle became pregnant two more times. She was hopeful, wanting, desperate. Both times Rochelle made it to her 5th month and in both cases the baby was born too early.

Each time, Rochelle's tiny precious baby was placed on her chest, breathed for about 30 minutes, and then slipped away. Our babies need iodine and minerals to live, thrive and stay alive.

Today, Rochelle is an aunt to her nieces and nephews, but she never fully experienced motherhood. Rochelle represents far too many women — bright, hopeful, full of longing — who never had the chance to raise their own children.

Their dreams of motherhood were silently sabotaged and stolen - most of them never understood the forces working against them. *Two cents a year* worth of iodine would have helped tremendously for Rochelle to have healthy pregnancies.

This is not just personal tragedy—it is patterned loss, written into the bodies of women across this country. What my cousin did not know is a severe iodine deficiency before and during pregnancy is associated with an increased risk of miscarriages, stillbirths, and infant mortality.

Toxins in Prenatal Vitamins

Analyses from U.S. researchers have raised alarms: only about **half** of prenatal vitamins sold in America contain iodine (Lee et al., 2017), and *fewer than half* contain meaningful amounts of choline—another nutrient essential for fetal memory and brain wiring (NIH ODS, 2025; Korsmo et al., 2019).

What's more, surveys have found detectable heavy metals like **lead and cadmium** in a *majority* of products, with a subset even exceeding *safe limits* (Gardener et al., 2025). Bottles look golden on the outside, but inside the capsules, the contents are gray, polluted, or insufficient.

When lead is in prenatal vitamins: exposure to lead damages a child's body and brain. It can cause:

- harm to the brain and nervous system
- slowed growth and development
- learning and behavior problems
- hearing and speech problems

Cadmium is Not Just a Contaminant

Cadmium is a toxin that can cross the placenta. This means a developing baby can be exposed *before it is even born*. Because the fetal stage is one of the most sensitive windows of human development, even small amounts of cadmium can interfere with organ formation, brain development, and long-term immune and hormonal health.

Continued exposure increases the risk of chronic diseases later in life. This is why clean prenatal vitamins — free of cadmium, lead, and other heavy metals — are essential for protecting both mother and child.

What this exposure can do: lower birth weight, slow growth, cause birth defects or developmental delays, and raise the risk of health problems that appear later in childhood or adulthood. Sometimes the harm is *not obvious right away* but shows up years later.

Those harms show up as real-life losses: lower IQ, trouble paying attention, and poor school performance. And it's not just for a little while — childhood *lead* exposure can leave lifelong damage - again making mothers believe it was her fault – something she did.

Heavy metals like cadmium, lead, and mercury cross the placenta and harm the developing brain.

Some clinicians suggest that iodine may support the body's ability to reduce certain toxic burdens. By now, you understand iodine's essential role in brain development and thyroid function. **But iodine does not work alone.**

Research shows that **a network of minerals and fat-soluble vitamins—including selenium, zinc, iron, calcium, and vitamins A, D, and E—act as the body's true defenders.**

- **Selenium** binds mercury and helps neutralize its harmful effects.
- **Zinc and iron** can reduce the absorption of cadmium and lead by competing for uptake in the gut.
- **Calcium** helps prevent stored lead from being released from bones during pregnancy. But don't take extra calcium that can turn to kidney stones. Instead, try boron and magnesium glycinate to help calcium absorb.
- **Vitamin C** and **glutathione-supporting nutrients** (which depend on selenium) aid the body's natural detoxification pathways.
- **Vitamins A, D, and E** protect cell membranes, support immune balance, and reduce oxidative stress during critical periods of brain development.

Before pregnancy—and throughout it—these nutrients form a **nutritional shield**, helping reduce toxic-metal burden and protect the developing brain long before birth.

Choline, too, is Essential

Choline builds cell membranes, fuels memory circuits, and wires the brain for resilience. Yet most prenatal vitamins still come up short.

Breastfeeding

And when a mother breastfeeds, she passes not only nutrients but also whatever toxins her body has stored. The CDC acknowledges that lead, for example, can transfer into breastmilk—though they emphasize that breastfeeding still offers far more benefits than risks, provided these toxic chemical exposures are reduced (CDC, 2024).

Make Sure Prenatal Vitamins are 3rd Party Tested

"Prenatal vitamins are regulated as dietary supplements, meaning the FDA does **not evaluate them for safety or effectiveness before they are sold to consumers."

This **does not mean supplements are unregulated** — they must meet labeling and manufacturing standards and cannot be misbranded or unsafe.

How Diagnosis Get Written

Too often the story unfolds like this: A child struggles to speak or focus.

- Lessons don't stick.
- Labels arrive: Nonverbal. ADHD. Learning disability. Autism spectrum. Behavioral disorder. Blind. Hearing impaired.
- A lifetime of medication follows.

But root causes go unnamed: missing iodine, low choline, weak selenium, gaps in minerals and vitamins - zinc, A, D, and E, and a nervous system trying to function while swimming through heavy metals and halogens. The diagnosis becomes a sentence, rather than a starting point for repair.

On a Personal Note

Sisters, when I was pregnant with my son, I saw various doctors and specialists. They ran every test, insurance paid for everything, and still—no one mentioned iodine, selenium and folate. I had gestational diabetes and severe polyhydramnios (too much fluid around the baby).

So, both my son and I remained iodine deficient. And when he entered school, he struggled and was placed in early intervention services at 9 months and special education classes at 3 years old.

But here is the real question - how is it possible that not a single obstetrician, gynecologist, family practitioner, and pediatrician—after years of college, residency, and medical practice—thought to check my iodine levels while I was pregnant or my children's iodine levels after they were born. Tell me, how is it no one knows about iodine?

My friends didn't know.

My mother didn't know.

My wise grandmothers didn't know.

The education system didn't teach it.

When lawmakers, medical institutions, corporations, and regulators ignore the laws of nature, the result is metabolic manipulation: women's wombs and breasts are targeted; girls' and boys' reproductive health and intelligence are impaired; the nation's mental health declines.

Without iodine, the body cannot excrete chemicals and toxins. So, they remain— circulating in the mother's bloodstream, embedding into her tissues, and crossing the placenta, depleting the new mother and the baby. Whatever the mother carries, the baby inherits.

That is why I am speaking to you now. I want my sisters to have the wisdom and knowledge I did not have—so you can have healthy pregnancies, safe deliveries, and children who thrive in school and in life.

Now that you understand iodine, I want to introduce you to the next missing nutrient—**Cod Liver Oil**—through a study I discovered during my research. It's time we reclaim wisdom.

Scientists *in other countries* studied pregnant women to see if cod liver oil (which contains healthy fats called EPA and DHA) could improve health during pregnancy.

Mothers Who Took Cod Liver Oil Had

- Lower blood sugar and better cholesterol levels.

- Lower hs-CRP, which means less inflammation.
- Lower HOMA-IR, which means better insulin sensitivity (their bodies used insulin more effectively).
- Fewer pregnancy complications than the group that didn't take cod liver oil.

What It Means

Cod liver oil helped:

- Keep blood sugar and fats in a healthy range
- Reduce swelling and inflammation
- Lower the chance of problems during pregnancy

Cod liver oil supported healthier pregnancies—helping mothers keep steadier blood sugar, face fewer complications, and possibly give their babies a stronger start.

Yet when nations skip iodine programs and ignore Mother Nature's gifts, clinicians aren't prompted to screen, counsel or treat our deficiency issues—and the diagnoses that could have been prevented go unseen.

It's time to flip the script.

1. Fill the proven gaps

- Iodine + Selenium: a duet. Iodine fuels the thyroid; selenium protects it and activates hormones.
- Choline: target ~450 mg/day in pregnancy (Korsmo et al., 2019).
- Vitamins A + D + E: food-first sources—cod liver oil and red palm oil.
- Cod liver oil contains omega-3 DHA: for brain health.
- Cod liver oil is not the same as fish oil. Cod comes from the sea and fish can come from a lake.

2. Bring the ocean home

Add sea-vegetables like nori, wakame, dulse or bladderwrack in moderation — or use reliable iodized salt from a country you know runs an iodine salt fortification program.

In the U.S., you may need to shop at Indian grocery stores (or online) for brands like Tata Iodized Salt — still one of the most affordable, reliable family-wide sources of iodine. Don't skip this simple step: it connects your kitchen to your birthright from the sea.

3. A Rice Warning

Cadmium: a silent poison our soils pass into food. It slips into bodies via rice grown in contaminated soils, seafood, organ meats, vegetables. The staple that fed generations may also carry the seeds of kidney failure, brittle bones, thyroid collapse, and clouded minds.

Arsenic, cadmium, and lead are natural parts of the earth. They are found in soil and water, so plants can take them in as they grow. Most foods have very small amounts, but some crops—especially grains like rice—can collect higher levels.

Over time, even low amounts of these metals can harm the body. They can raise the risk of *cancer, damage the brain and nerves, and cause learning or developmental problems,* especially in babies and children.

When scientists talk about "Southeastern U.S. rice," they are mostly talking about rice grown in *Arkansas, Louisiana, Mississippi, and parts of Texas and Missouri.* These states grow a lot of rice, and some of the highest heavy-metal levels have been found in rice from this region.

Most of the rice we eat contains arsenic, cadmium, and lead whether it's brown rice, white rice and infant rice. Brown rice generally has higher arsenic (because the bran retains more) compared to white rice. To lower the toxic levels, rinse well prior to cooking and diversify grains to lower arsenic exposure.

Tests were conducted to identify three types of rice consistently lower in total heavy metals: *California-grown rice (California, USA), Thai jasmine rice (Thailand), and Indian basmati rice (India).* "Lower" does **not** mean "none". Any rice will likely contain some amount of heavy metals because of soil, water, and growing conditions.

Breastmilk will always be the gold standard. You don't need to replace it — you strengthen it by strengthening *you.* Research from the CDC (2024) and ACOG (2021) shows that a mother's mineral status directly shapes the quality of her milk.

Mothers and mothers-to-be, staying healthy today takes intentional effort. We live in a world filled with environmental chemicals and hidden nutrient gaps, and every day you are making choices that protect your family's future. My goal here is simple: to guide you, support you, and help you nourish both yourself and your child with wisdom and ease.

Eat Rice in Moderation

In the U.S., we eat a lot of rice—fried rice, Thai rice, rice cakes, rice noodles, sushi rice, and even infant rice cereal. Rice shows up on our plates, in our snacks, in school lunches, and in baby food.

Black Rice or Wild Rice

Black rice *can* contain arsenic, lead, or cadmium, but:

- Levels are **lower than brown rice**
- Levels are **lower than most white rice**
- Heavy-metal content depends on where it's grown

Black rice has **more antioxidants** (anthocyanins), which offer some protection — but the grain still absorbs arsenic from the soil the same way other rice varieties do.

Wild rice is a seed from aquatic grass, not a true rice grain. Because of this, it does not accumulate arsenic the way white, brown, or black rice do.

- *Lowest arsenic levels*
- Very low heavy metals
- High in minerals and antioxidants

Wild rice is one of the cleanest, safest alternatives for families.

Best Method to Lower Heavy Metals In Rice

Rinsing the rice before cooking can reduce a small amount of surface arsenic (and a bit of cadmium), but the effect is limited. Rinsing removes about 10–20% of arsenic that is on the outside of the grain.

It does **not** remove the arsenic stored *inside* the grain (especially in brown rice). So rinsing is helpful, but it's not enough by itself. Use the excess-water method to drain additional heavy metals, similar to cooking pasta:

This method can remove **up to 50–60%** of arsenic in some white rice varieties. Brown rice will remove less, but still more than rinsing alone.

1. Rinse rice well.
2. Cook the rice in 5–6 cups of water per 1 cup of rice.
3. When the rice is done, **drain the extra water**.
4. Fluff and serve.

That means whatever is in the rice—good or harmful—quickly becomes part of our bodies and our children's bodies. This is why choosing the *right* kind of grain matters. Better grain options that usually contain lower heavy metals are millet, quinoa and oats.

Important for Mothers

Infant rice cereal is one of the **highest arsenic-containing** foods for babies. Alternatives include:

- Oatmeal
- Quinoa cereal
- Millet cereal

Toxic Titanium Dioxide in Our Food

Titanium Dioxide. Banned in Europe as a food additive because of safety concerns (EFSA, 2022). They worry it might damage DNA, especially in tiny (nano) form. Nano form" means super tiny pieces—so small you can't see them even with a regular microscope.

This is a bright white chemical used to make foods look whiter. It's often found as the white outer coating on chewy candy and gum, and it's the white powder sprinkled on donuts to make them look brighter and more perfect.

Common Foods That May Contain Titanium Dioxide

- **Chewy candies** (like Skittles, Starburst, Mentos)
- **Gum** (many brands use a white coating)
- **Powdered donuts** (the bright white sugar on top)
- **Icing and frostings** (to make the color look brighter)
- **Sprinkles** (especially white or rainbow sprinkles)
- **Coffee creamers** (to make them look smoother and whiter)
- **White sauces** (some brands use it to make sauces look more "creamy")
- **Processed snacks** (like snack cakes and some cereals)
- **Store-bought baked goods** (to give them a bright, clean look)

A few years ago, I attended a meeting at work on a day when I was tired. The presenter happened to be seated right beside me, so heavy eyelids were not an option. I asked a colleague for gum, thinking it would help me stay alert. She handed me two small, white square pieces, which I popped into my mouth.

Moments later, I began coughing—violently. I wasn't nodding off anymore; I was struggling to breathe, right next to the presenter. Then it hit me: *white-coated gum*. Titanium dioxide!!!!

I immediately stood up and rushed to the restroom, coughing until I expelled what felt like the entire coating into the toilet. In that moment, I made a decision: To pay closer attention to everything even if I feel tired.

A Mother's Closing Prayer

Let the womb be a sanctuary, not a storage unit for toxins. Sabotage ends here.

CHAPTER 7 BIBLIOGRAPHY

1. **American College of Obstetricians and Gynecologists.** *Committee Opinion No. 803: Reducing Prenatal Exposure to Toxic Environmental Agents. Obstetrics & Gynecology* 137, no. 1 (2021): e1–e12.
2. **Bennett, J. P., et al.** "Heavy Metals in Wild Rice from North-Central Wisconsin."
3. **Cianchetta, S., et al.** "Perchlorate Transport and Inhibition of the Sodium-Iodide Symporter (NIS)." *Toxicology and Applied Pharmacology* 243 (2010): 58–65.
4. **Centers for Disease Control and Prevention.** *Lead and Breastfeeding.* Atlanta: CDC, 2024.
5. **European Food Safety Authority.** *Opinion on the Safety of Titanium Dioxide (E171) as a Food Additive.* European Commission, 2022.
6. **Gardener, H., et al.** "Heavy Metals and Phthalate Contamination in Prenatal Vitamins." *American Journal of Clinical Nutrition* (2025).
7. **Health.com.** "Which Rice Types Have the Most Arsenic and Heavy Metals?" *Health.com*, 2025.
8. **Korsmo, H. W., et al.** "Choline: Exploring the Growing Science on Its Benefits for Moms and Babies." *Nutrients* 11, no. 8 (2019): 1823.
9. **Lee, S. Y., et al.** "Iodine Contents in Prenatal Vitamins in the United States." *Thyroid* 27, no. 9 (2017): 1170–1175.
10. **Lisco, G., et al.** "Interference on Iodine Uptake and Human Thyroid Function by Environmental Pollutants." *International Journal of Molecular Sciences* 21, no. 20 (2020): 7503.

11. **National Institutes of Health, Office of Dietary Supplements.** *Dietary Supplements and Life Stages: Pregnancy.* NIH, 2025.
12. **NutritionFacts.org.** "Which Rice Has the Least Amount of Arsenic (Black, Brown, Red, White, or Wild?)." *NutritionFacts.org*, 2020.
13. **Patrick, L.** "Lead Toxicity, a Review of the Literature. Part I: Exposure, Evaluation, and Treatment." *Alternative Medicine Review* 11, no. 1 (2006): 2–22.
14. **Rayman, M. P.** "Selenium and Human Health." *The Lancet* 379, no. 9822 (2012): 1256–1268.
15. **Sarkar, R. D., et al.** "Health Risk from Toxic Metals in Wild Rice Grown in the Upper Peninsula of Michigan." *Applied Sciences* 12, no. 6 (2022): 2937.
16. **Sonawane, B. R., M. Nordberg, G. F. Nordberg, and G. W. Lucier.** "Placental Transfer of Cadmium in Rats: Influence of Dose and Gestational Age." *Environmental Health Perspectives* 12, no. 1 (1975): 97–102.
17. **Teas, J., S. Vena, D. L. Cone, and M. Irhimeh.** "Seaweed Consumption as a Protective Factor in Breast Cancer: Proof of Principle." *Journal of Applied Phycology* 25 (2013): 771–779.
18. **U.S. Food and Drug Administration.** *Dietary Supplements: Tips for Women.* FDA, last modified March 22, 2023. https://www.fda.gov/consumers/womens-health-topics/dietary-supplements-tips-women
19. **Velasco, I., S. C. Bath, and M. P. Rayman.** "Iodine as an Essential Nutrient during the First 1000 Days of Life." *Nutrients* 10, no. 3 (2018): 290.

CHAPTER 8

PLACENTA TO PRISON PIPELINE

The United States loves to call itself the "land of opportunity." Yet behind the headlines and the flag waving lies a disturbing truth: millions of Americans cannot read, cannot think clearly, and cannot function with the mental clarity a civilized nation requires.

The Black community, once celebrated for its genius —inventions, innovations, breakthroughs, artistry, and leadership — now sees generation after generation of children robbed of that same brilliance. Not because of lack of talent, but because of the silent theft of the very minerals that build intelligence.

When iodine and selenium disappear from the diet, when mothers receive prenatal vitamins full of promises but empty of power, the consequences appear in classrooms, courtrooms, and homes. What we call "illiteracy" is not a mystery. It is a mineral tragedy.

From Empty Plates to Prison Gates

America talks about crime as though it begins in alleyways. But it often begins in the womb.

A child growing inside a mother deficient in iodine and selenium begins life already disadvantaged. By school age, that child struggles to focus, process information, or manage emotions.

Teachers call it behavior.

Doctors call it disorder.

Society calls it failure.

But what it truly is — is deficiency.

This is a pipeline not from school to prison, but from **placenta to prison**.

For generations, Black children — naturally brilliant — have been mislabeled "slow" and funneled into special education.

Adolescence brings discipline instead of guidance, detention instead of opportunity, and handcuffs instead of hope.

Not because Black children are less capable — but because their brains were robbed of the raw materials needed for intelligence. Iodine is the brain's battery. Without it, cognition cannot ignite. A malnourished brain cannot read, cannot reason, cannot rise.

The Literacy Numbers America Hides

The official data claims America is 89% literate. But the truth is far darker.

- **334 million people live in America. 130 million adults** ages 16–74 cannot read beyond a 5th-grade level.
- **50 million foreign-born residents,** mostly from iodized-salt nations, maintain higher literacy. So, I won't count them in the literacy count.
- That leaves **285 million U.S.-born Americans** whose literacy should reflect American schooling.

But the statistics hide millions of struggling children in kindergarten through the 9th grade:

- speech delays
- learning disabilities
- ADHD
- autism spectrum disorder
- comprehension difficulties
- undiagnosed reading challenges

Conservatively, **10–20 million children** fall into these categories. When you include these children, the true picture emerges:

America's actual literacy rate is closer to 50.9%, not 89%.

Half the nation cannot read.

Half the nation cannot navigate a world built on words.

Half the nation is mentally underpowered — before adulthood.

This crisis did not appear on its own.

It began with **mineral deficiency, toxic food,** and **unsupported brain development**.

We sent our children into battle *without* armor.

The Real-Life State of Emergency

I witness the crisis everyday firsthand:

- Children who cannot remember their home address or their parent's phone number.
- First-graders with panic attacks dismissed as "funny."
- Teachers overwhelmed, classrooms collapsing.
- Parents confused, handed only prescriptions and labels.
- Younger toddler students in special needs classes need careful and consistent watch because they eat cardboard, plastic, and sometimes their own feces.

Pica is a condition where a person has a persistent urge to eat non-food substances that have no nutritional value.

Common examples of pica

People with pica may crave or eat:

- Dirt or clay
- Chalk
- Ice (a common form called *pagophagia*)
- Paper
- Soap
- Ashes
- Hair
- Paint chips
- Starch (laundry starch or cornstarch)

Why pica happens

Pica is often a **signal of deficiency**, not a behavior problem. It is commonly linked to:

- *Iron deficiency*
- *Zinc deficiency*
- *Iodine and other mineral deficiencies*
- Pregnancy (increased mineral demand)

- Childhood growth phases
- Chronic malnutrition or food insecurity

Why it's dangerous

Eating non-food items can lead to:

- Lead or toxin exposure
- Intestinal blockages
- Infections or parasites
- Worsening nutrient deficiencies

Pica is the body's cry for missing minerals. When essential nutrients are absent, the brain drives a person to seek substances that resemble earth, minerals, or texture—mistaking them for nourishment.

The Spiral of Dysfunction

When the brain starves, dysfunction spreads:

- Teens are angry, anxious, disconnected from themselves—expressed through their confusion, decisions and their behavior.
- School shootings
- Parental neglect and tragedy
- Little ones left unsupervised in the backseat of hot cars where they died; others mauled to death by dogs or left at home alone.
- Child-on-child violence
- Spouse killings
- Homicide-suicides, molestation, murders, road rage, cycles of abuse, and suicidal ideation spread like wildfire through communities.

The jail holds the accused —
but the iodine-withholder is never charged.

Zombie Nation

Seventy-eight years without adequate iodine has produced a nation on autopilot:

- Brain fog

- Memory loss
- Alzheimer's (7.2 million seniors today)
- Opioid collapse
- Emotional numbness
- Cognitive exhaustion

A mentally compromised nation cannot thrive.

Yet the government spends billions on prisons — instead of pennies on iodized salt.

Let Me Show You Iodine Across the Americas

Andean Mothers

Remember the 1830s study in Andes, South America where the French chemist, Boussingault discovered iodine and stated:

"If the people lack iodine because they are far from the sea...then add iodine to the salt. Give iodine to everyone."

In the Andes, iodine deficiency did not just affect statistics—it affected mothers.

Studies in severely deficient regions revealed widespread maternal hypothyroidism and babies born into a world already dimmed by scarcity. Some infants developed cretinism. Many more carried hidden losses—lower IQ, impaired hearing, delayed language—losses that would be blamed on culture, poverty, or fate, when the root cause was a missing micronutrient.

Then something radical happened: prevention became a priority.

National Iodine Deficiency Prevention Programs in Latin America

Country	National Iodization Program (Year)	Government Support	Monitoring Capacity
Argentina	1993	Ministry of Health	National Program
Bolivia	1984	Ministry of Health	National Program
Brazil	1992	Ministry of Health	National Program
Chile	1995	Ministry of Health	National Program
Colombia	1993	Ministry of Health	National Program
Costa Rica	1998	Ministry of Health	National Program
Cuba	1993	Ministry of Health	National Program

Country	National Iodization Program (Year)	Government Support	Monitoring Capacity
Dominican Republic	1999	Ministry of Health	National Program
Ecuador	1984	Ministry of Health	National Program
El Salvador	1993	Ministry of Health	INCAP
Guatemala	1992	Ministry of Health	National Program
Haiti	2000	Ministry of Health	Limited
Honduras	1993	Ministry of Health	INCAP
Mexico	1996	Ministry of Health	National Program
Nicaragua	1993	Ministry of Health	INCAP
Panama	1997	Ministry of Health	National Program
Paraguay	1991	Ministry of Health	National Program
Peru	1984	Ministry of Health	National Program
Uruguay	1990	Ministry of Health	National Program
Venezuela	1992	Ministry of Health	National Program

Source: Adapted from Pretell and Pearce (2024).

NOTE: <u>National Programs</u> protect iodine through law, monitoring, and enforcement; <u>INCAP</u> provides shared regional scientific oversight; and <u>Limited</u> programs lack sufficient monitoring, placing long-term iodine sufficiency at risk.

Where monitoring is limited, memory fades. Where monitoring is shared and sustained, intelligence is protected.

Iodized oil protected high-risk populations quickly, and iodized salt became the long-term shield. But the greatest shift was not only in iodine—it was in **commitment**: monitoring, enforcement, education, and public messaging that treated iodine as a national responsibility.

Latin America proves what is possible when nations choose protection over neglect. With over 90% of households consuming iodized salt, children across the region now show optimal iodine status, not by accident—but by design.

This success did not come from hope or individual choice; it came from **government commitment, monitoring, and public education**. And the lesson is clear: iodine sufficiency is not a one-time victory. To my Latin American neighbors-this is why you have the beautiful brain capacity to speak at least two or more languages.

Canadians
Your natural iodine access has spared you much of the crisis in the U.S.

Where vigilance remains, intelligence rises.

From the Alps to Africa, from Central Asia to East Asia, the pattern repeats: when iodine is monitored, minds flourish; when it is ignored, generations pay the price. Iodine programs must be **guarded**, **measured**, and **defended** across generations.

Where oversight fades, deficiency returns quietly. Progress is fragile—but prevention is simple when leadership remembers its responsibility.

The Plot to Biologically Destroy Black America

When I say "Black," I speak of the Original Originals—the people whose melanin was designed by the sun itself, whose cells remember iodine, selenium, and sea minerals, whose brilliance shaped nations long before nations had names.

Some call us Chosen, Hebrew, Olmecs and the people in the Bible. Some say we are the rightful inheritors of a stolen story. But beneath every title lies one unchanging truth: we are the foundation.

The blueprint.

The root from which genius grows.

But for 78 years and counting, Black Americans have suffered a silent biological assault:

- Withheld iodine
- Toxic potassium bromates in food
- Nutrient-depleted soil
- Chemical additives in food that are banned elsewhere
- High miscarriage rates
- Rising infertility
- Postpartum collapse
- Generational cognitive decline

Four generations deficient and the patterns are the proof: This is not genetic. This is nutritional sabotage.

American Tax Payer Dollars Fund Global Literacy Abroad

American tax dollars have literally financed Iodized-Salt Systems abroad beyond our borders. U.S. funds have long funded literacy drives in other lands: in Lebanon, USAID's multi-phase QITABI (now QITABI 3) scales early reading nationwide; in Central Asia USAID has financed foundational-skills programs in the *Kyrgyzstan* Republic (Okuu Keremet!), *Tajikistan* (Quality Reading Project and national EGRAs), and *Uzbekistan* (Education for Excellence with national EGRA/EGMA follow-ups), while regional initiatives include *Kazakhstan*.

Across Africa, American funded early-grade reading projects have reached Kenya (Tusome), Tanzania (Tusome Pamoja), Uganda (SHRP/LARA), Rwanda (Soma Umenye), Senegal (Lecture Pour Tous/RELIT), Liberia (Read Liberia), Ghana (EGR Program), Nigeria (Northern Education Initiative & EGRA), Malawi (Early Grade Reading Activity), Zambia (Let's Read), Mozambique (Vamos Ler!), Mali (SIRA/ Doniya Taabolo), and others.

Programs funded by American taxpayers have raised literacy and intelligence abroad, yet America's own children have quietly declined. The nation did not merely stagnate—it regressed. We went back in time. Back more than 200 years.

Back to the conditions that gripped the Alps in 1788, when a mineral-starved population suffered widespread cognitive impairment. What Europe once called a tragedy of history; America allowed it to become a modern reality.

What does that mean in practice? It means American tax dollars have literally financed iodized-salt systems abroad—not just buying salt for families but building entire national infrastructures for iodine delivery.

Through USAID, in partnership with UNICEF, the Iodine Global Network (IGN), and the Global Alliance for Improved Nutrition (GAIN), the U.S. has paid for potassium iodate supplies, iodization machinery, training for salt producers, quality-control laboratories, and public-health monitoring across Africa, the Middle East, and Central Asia.

In Lebanon, Ethiopia, Madagascar, Kenya, Nigeria, and the Central Asian republics, these U.S.-backed programs ensure mothers and children overseas receive the very nutrient our own families have been denied.

We built a portion of the world's iodine systems.

We built a portion of the world's literacy systems.

But our country abandoned us!!

The United States protects every nation's brain — except its own.

This is not an oversight.

It is a **policy slaughter** that began in 1948.

This is the double standard of global health:

The hand that feeds the world iodine lives in an iodine famine.

Our biology was targeted, our heritage undermined, and our dignity assaulted—not by chance, but by neglect and design. Whole communities were left nutritionally unguarded while systems moved on without them.

Today, disproportionately, millions of Black and Hispanic brothers and sisters sit behind bars, casualties of generations denied the minerals that support cognition, impulse control, learning, and clarity. At the same time, labor pipelines increasingly rely on populations whose brains were protected in their countries by iodine-sufficient public-health programs.

This is not a story about immigrants versus citizens—it is a warning about what happens when a nation fails to defend the neurological inheritance of its own people. When intelligence is not protected at the beginning of life, entire populations become expendable in the machinery of modern society.

So, when you find yourself asking why certain doors felt heavier to open—why effort did not always yield equal return—understand this: what you are witnessing is not individual weakness. It is collective injury.

When learning in school felt difficult, or maybe when a relationship ended tragically, or when work or school demanded more effort than they should, now you have context. And once you see it in yourself, you begin to recognize it in others as well. Recognizing it is the first step toward restoration. This understanding does not assign blame towards our people; it restores clarity.

The Path Forward

We cannot wait another seventy-eight years for a government that has already turned on us. The solution must arise from homes, mothers, fathers, families, and communities:

We must build coalitions — I dream of a *Planet Oversight Coalition* — a global circle of guardians who refuse to let any family slip through the cracks again. Because the home we overlook today may be the very home that births tomorrow's tragedy. Prevention is protection, and protection is how we safeguard the future.

Health is wealth.

Nourishment is freedom.

And a nation that remembers this will rise again

CHAPTER 8 BIBLIOGRAPHY

1. **USAID Global Education & Early Grade Reading Reports**
   U.S. Agency for International Development. *Global Education and Early Grade Reading Program Reports: QITABI & QITABI 3 (Lebanon); Okuu Keremet! (Kyrgyz Republic); Quality Reading Project and EGRA (Tajikistan); Education for Excellence (Uzbekistan); Regional Education Initiatives (Kazakhstan); and African Early Grade Reading Programs, including Tusome (Kenya), Tusome Pamoja (Tanzania), SHRP/LARA (Uganda), Soma Umenye (Rwanda), Lecture Pour Tous/RELIT (Senegal), Read Liberia, EGR (Ghana), Northern Education Initiative & EGRA (Nigeria), Early Grade Reading Activity (Malawi), Let's Read (Zambia), Vamos Ler! (Mozambique), and SIRA/Doniya Taabolo (Mali).* USAID Evaluation and Performance Reports, 2020–2024.

2. **UNICEF, Iodine Global Network & GAIN Partnership Reports**
   UNICEF and Iodine Global Network. *Universal Salt Iodization and Iodine Deficiency Elimination Partnership Reports.* 2023–2024.
   Global Alliance for Improved Nutrition (GAIN). *Program Summaries on Universal Salt Iodization Initiatives.* Various years.

3. **USAID Health & Nutrition Portfolios**
   U.S. Agency for International Development. *Health and Nutrition Portfolio Reports: Lebanon, Ethiopia, Madagascar, Kenya, Nigeria, and Central Asia.* Various years.

4. **Mannar & Dunn — Achieving Universal Salt Iodization**
   Mannar, M. G. V., and John T. Dunn. *Achieving Universal Salt Iodization: I. Background.* Iodine Global Network / World Health Organization, 2009. https://files.givewell.org/files/DWDA%202009/Interventions/Iodine/Achieving%20Universal%20Salt%20Iodization.pdf.

5. **Ingram & Blum — U.S. Foreign Aid Architecture**
   Ingram, George, and Walter Blum. *Institutional Architecture of U.S. Foreign Aid.* Washington, DC: Brookings Institution, 2017. https://www.brookings.edu/wp-content/uploads/2017/08/global-20170731-blum-georgeingram-brief-31.pdf.

6. **USAID Overview (Congressional Research Service)**
   U.S. Agency for International Development. *U.S. Agency for International Development: An Overview.* Congressional Research Service Report No. IF10261, 2025. https://crsreports.congress.gov/product/pdf/IF/IF10261.

7. **Executive Order 10973**
   United States. *Executive Order No. 10973: Administration of Foreign Assistance and Related Functions.* 26 Fed. Reg. 10749 (November 3, 1961). The American Presidency Project.

8. **Foreign Assistance Act of 1961** United States. *Foreign Assistance Act of 1961.* Pub. L. No. 87-195, 75 Stat. 424 (1961).

9. **Pretell & Pearce — Elimination of iodine deficiency in the Americas (2024)**
   Pretell, Eduardo A., and Elizabeth N. Pearce. "A History of the Elimination of Iodine Deficiency Disorders in the Americas: A Dramatic Achievement and Lessons Learned." *The Journal of Nutrition* 154, no. 12 (2024): 3856–3867. https://doi.org/10.1016/j.tjnut.2024.10.009.

10. **Pretell et al. — Public health triumph in the Americas**
    Pretell, Eduardo A., Elizabeth N. Pearce, Sergio A. Moreno, Omar Dary, Roland Kupka, and Michael B. Zimmermann. "Elimination of Iodine Deficiency Disorders from the Americas: A Public Health Triumph." *The Lancet Diabetes & Endocrinology* 5, no. 6 (2017): 412–414. https://doi.org/10.1016/S2213-8587(17)30034-7.

11. **WHO/UNICEF/ICCIDD — Universal Salt Iodization framework**
    World Health Organization, UNICEF, and ICCIDD. *Assessment of Iodine Deficiency Disorders and Monitoring Their Elimination: A Guide for Programme Managers.* 3rd ed. Geneva: World Health Organization, 2007.

CHAPTER 9

THE KEEPERS OF THE SPOON

(A lesson from 100 years ago)

A Daily Ritual in the Classroom

Picture a chilly morning in the 1920s or '30s. Children in wool sweaters shuffle into class. A teacher stands by a tray of small cups and spoons, amber bottle in hand. One by one, students swallow a spoonful of cod liver oil, make a face and continue on with their day. This simple ritual protected an entire generation.

The Problem Schools Were Fighting

In northern cities, children faced widespread deficiencies:

Too Little Sunlight → Vitamin D Deficiency

Long winters, coal smoke, factory smog, and cramped housing blocked UV light. **Results:** rickets, bowed legs, fragile bones, delayed growth.

Thin Diets → Low Vitamin A & Omega-3s

Families lived on cheap starches. Fish, butter, eggs, and produce were scarce. **Results:** poor immunity, night-vision problems, slow healing.

Schools became the front line of defense.

Why Teachers Became Healers

Clinics were scarce. Mothers worked long hours. Many families couldn't afford a doctor.

Schools Could Reach Every Child

Teachers and school nurses:

- Distributed cod liver oil
- Checked teeth and eyesight
- Taught hygiene
- Tracked growth

It was **public health through routine**, not prescriptions.

Girls Often Lined Up First

Photos show long lines of girls because:

- Many schools were sex-segregated
- Educators understood that **healthy girls → healthy future pregnancies → healthy next generation**

A girl carries all her future eggs at birth. Nourishing her is nourishing tomorrow's children.

A Movement Across Nations

Scandinavia & North Atlantic

Cod liver oil was a household staple. Schools normalized it.

Britain (WWII Era)

Despite rationing, the government provided cod liver oil and orange juice to children and pregnant women.

United States & Canada

Schools and settlement houses used cod liver oil to fight rickets and winter illness in industrial cities.

It was **prevention**, not luxury.

Why the Ritual Faded

By the 1940s–1960s:

- Vitamin D was added to milk
- Diets improved

- Housing and sunlight exposure increased
- Pediatric medicine expanded

But the wisdom disappeared.

What Those Teachers Already Knew

Without biochemical jargon, teachers observed:

- Fewer bowed legs
- Stronger immune systems
- Clearer night vision
- Steadier energy
- Healthier growth

They saw **stronger, brighter children** — the goal of every generation.

Möller's: A Spoonful of Life

Since 1854, Möller's Cod Liver Oil has symbolized nourishment.
On the bottle of the cod liver oil label you'll find:

- **A first-aid cross** → immune strength
- **A brain icon** → intelligence
- **Eye symbols** → vision
- **A jumping child** → vitality

Each symbol speaks a mother's language:
protect the whole child. Sometimes mothers needed reminders. The bottle was a silent ally.

What Cod Liver Oil Carried

The Essential Nutrients

- **Vitamin D** → strong bones, straight legs, proper growth
- **Vitamin A** → immunity, eyesight, tissue repair
- **DHA (Omega-3)** → brain formation, memory, emotional balance
- **Healthy fats** → metabolism, heart health

Prenatal Readiness

A well-nourished girl grows into a well-nourished mother.

The nutrients she receives today echo into the lives of the children she will carry tomorrow.

Dated European Cod Liver Oil Advertisements

In the 1940s–50s, European cod liver oil advertisements emphasized:

1. "Take Cod Liver Oil to build the perfect-sized head and straight legs."
   While American children struggled with macrocephaly, scoliosis, and rickets.
2. "Take Cod Liver Oil to prevent future mental breakdown; prevent crooked teeth."
   American children faced overcrowded teeth, braces, and rising mental health crises.
3. "Take Cod Liver Oil for superhuman immune system, beautiful hair, balanced hormones, sharp brain function."
4. "Take Cod Liver Oil to regulate cholesterol naturally."
5. "Take Cod Liver oil for proper brain development during pregnancy."

Europe understood the power of nourishing the mother to nourish the child. Later, in homes where cod liver oil and iodized salt were cherished, children:

- Learned faster
- Saw better
- Stood taller
- Spoke multiple languages
- Excelled academically
- Outgrew winter illnesses

Brain & Mental Health

Low vitamin D status at birth has been associated in research with increased risk of:

- ADHD
- Autism spectrum traits

- Schizophrenia
- Mood disorders

The blueprint is written early—**in the womb**.

Keepers of the Spoon

Why We Must Bring the Ocean Home

Today's children face pressures unknown to previous generations:

- Air pollution
- Traffic-corridor toxins
- Perchlorates that block iodine uptake
- Ultra-processed foods
- Indoor lifestyles with little sunlight
- Widespread nutrient deficiencies

The environment has changed. The nourishment must be intentional.

Our Solution

When we cannot reach the seaside, **we strategically bring the sea and earth home**:

- Cod liver oil
- Seaweed
- Iodized salt
- Selenium
- Red palm oil

We are not reinventing the wheel.
We are remembering.

Nutrition Without Meaning Became Compliance Without Wisdom

Norway kept the ritual alive.
America drifted.

America fortified foods—but lost the **story**, the **ritual**, and the **purpose**. And children paid the price through:

- Brittle winters of illness
- Weakened immunity
- Preventable learning challenges

Nutrition without meaning became compliance without wisdom.

A Simple Daily Blueprint

- **Feed the Thyroid:** Iodine + selenium
- **Feed the Brain:** DHA
- **Feed the Eyes & Skin:** Vitamins A + E (cod liver oil, red palm oil)
- **Feed the Future:**

  - Nourish girls → nourish generations
  - Nourish boys → protect future fathers

This is elemental—not complicated.

Closing Blessing: The Return of the Spoon

A spoonful of life since 1854—not as advertisement, but as heritage.
All components of the firmament has mothered humanity since the beginning.
Remembering this wisdom is why our grandmothers knew what to do:
Find what is missing—and feed it.
Let the final message be simple and sovereign:
Nourish the womb.
Nourish the child.
Nourish the future.
Women and teachers were once the **keepers of the spoon** because they were the keepers of the children.
They did not wait for permission to protect the next generation.
What they did with a spoon,
we can now do with knowledge—
Together, we can help every child
stand tall, think fast, and live long.

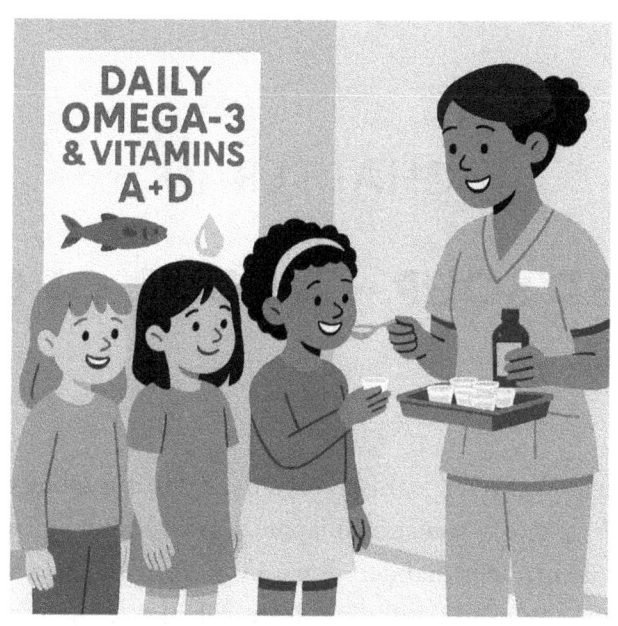
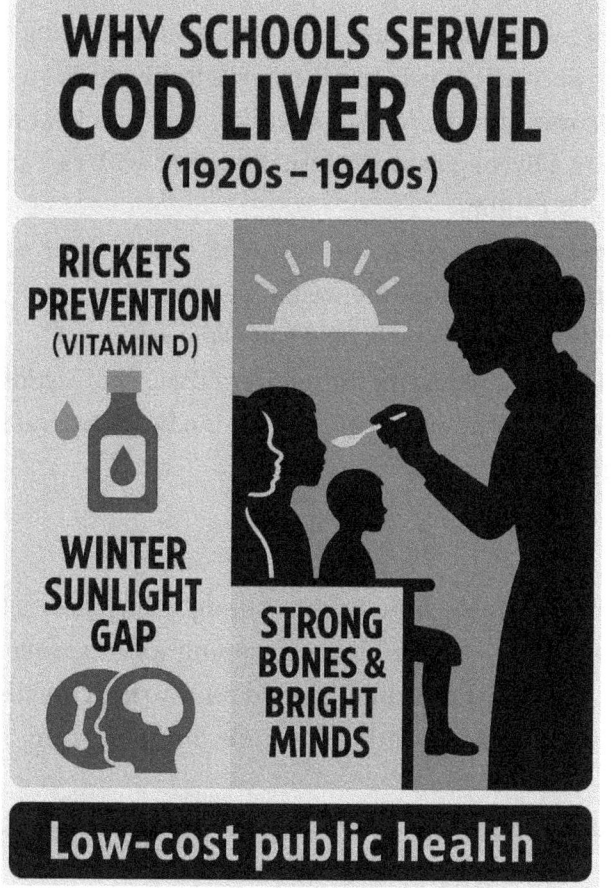

Mother's Wit Approved.

CHAPTER 10

SEAWEED SOUP – A BOWL OF GENIUS

If this book has a last prayer, it is this: return the sea to our tables and the wisdom to our kitchens. *Miyeokguk*—wakame in Japan, seaweed soup in Korea—is more than a recipe. It is a medicine chest handed down by Korean mothers and grandmothers who know what the ocean gives: iodine, iron, calcium, magnesium and a river of nutrients that help a new mother regenerate after birth and feed her newborn's brain.

In Korea, *miyeokguk* is not just food—it's a longstanding tradition that has served generations well. After birth, families serve it three times a day for a month so the mother can recover quickly, rebuild strength, and pass vital nutrients including iodine onto her baby. Miyeokguk soup is usually served with rice and other vegetables for a complete meal for mom.

Tradition insists mom stays home, rest, and be cared for so she can focus on healing and breastfeeding without the weight of work or errands. This is care made visible: a community saying, *"We will hold you while you mend."*

This simple bowl is a blueprint for recovery that other nations have kept while we were left out. But this is how we realign. This is a beautiful tradition we can adopt with the highest gratitude.

Wisdom in a bowl

Picture elders whose eyes shine with wisdom, telling stories that stitch families together. Picture a mother, wrapped in care, sipping warm seaweed soup, rebuilding her strength, and passing elements of mind and body to her child through breastmilk. Imagine children who grow up with full minds, not hungering for what the earth freely gives.

That is the future *miyeokguk* promises—not because soup is magic, but because when you feed the body what it needs, brilliance follows.

So, this is where *stolen intellect* and illiteracy end, and the *Genius Revolution* begins: at the table. We will stop waiting on broken policy. We will feed our babies, honor our elders, and teach our people how to reclaim health.

Bring seaweed to your pot. Teach your sister, your neighbor, your grandmother. Keep the great-grandparents here. Keep their stories alive and their minds sharp.

If you wish to end this book with one act, let it be this: make a pot of *miyeokguk*, share it, and make sure the next generation is born into a home that knows how to nourish a healthy genius. Feed the sea back into our bodies—and watch a nation remember how to think.

Korea's 21-day postpartum period, *samchil-il*, treats *recovery* like the emergency it is. *Miyeokguk* is the daily remedy: dried seaweed simmered into broth, often with beef or seafood for protein. It's a dense, natural source of iodine (for thyroid and energy), iron (to rebuild after blood loss), and calcium (to strengthen bones as the baby draws what it needs). Seaweed soup also brings vitamin K, magnesium, folate, fiber, and hydration—everything a mother needs to heal and nourish her infant.

A ritual of gratitude and protection

Beyond nutrients, *miyeokguk* carries care. Eating it is a ritual of gratitude and protection: mothers, grandmothers, and neighbors prepare pots and bring them to new families. That ritual—consistent, communal, intentional feeding—adds a psychological and cultural layer to the physical recovery.

Warm soup, reliable nutrients, and steady attention: that combination helps a mother recover faster and keeps both her and her baby stronger.

Miyeokguk reminds us that the ocean and the land already give us what we need. It's not superstition—it's science woven with tradition. For mothers everywhere, it's a model: feed the body well after birth, support the breasts, mend the blood, and surround the mother with care. That's how postpartum *recovery* replaces postpartum *depression*.

For the first three to six weeks after childbirth, leaving the house is discouraged. Give yourself and your newborn time to heal and build a strong immune system. Seaweed soup shows up at every meal for about a month. In countries where people eat seaweed, they have some of the highest IQs in the world.

Birthday Ritual: Miyeokguk (Seaweed Soup)

In Korea, *miyeokguk*—seaweed soup—is served to honor a mother's labor and love. Each year on their birthday, Koreans mark the day they were born with a warm bowl of this nourishing soup. It's often called **"birthday soup."** Birthday Soup: a yearly reminder to thank mothers and to nourish the next generation.

A Symbol of Motherhood

Miyeokguk soup serves as a ritual recognizing a mother's sacrifice, honoring the body that carried life, and reminding the family to feed recovery with care.

The Legend

One popular story says early observers noticed whales eating seaweed after giving birth, inspiring the belief that seaweed supports a new mother's recovery.

Whether legend or lesson, the practice took root: seaweed soup became a trusted part of the postpartum diet for rebuilding strength and nourishment. Lessons are everywhere. They are all around us.

Note:

Sea vegetables alone (miyeokguk can be made without meat and still remain medicinal).

The healing power of miyeokguk comes from the sea, not the meat. Protein is supportive—but **minerals are the medicine.**

CHAPTER 11

THE GIFT OF A WELL-NOURISHED MIND

The Gift of Intelligence - Intelligence is the ability to understand, to solve, to create, to adapt. It is curiosity stretching toward answers.

Genius is intelligence set aflame—extraordinary intellectual power, expressed in creativity, invention, and vision.

IQ—intelligence quotient—is only one way to measure it. True genius often escapes tests. It lives in how we solve problems, nurture our children, build communities, and imagine a future beyond what we see.

"The earth, the air, the ocean, and the sun—Behold, the divine cosmic recipe for intelligence, sound mind, health and longevity. When wisdom fuels genius, greatness is born, and with it comes freedom."

Beholding Human Potential

When I meet people from around the world, I marvel at their genius, their ability to speak multiple languages, variety of talents, skills, and expressions of creativity. I always ask the same question: *"Where are you from?"*

The answer often speaks volumes about both health and destiny. If they live by a toxic river or lake, I sometimes hear stories of rare cancers. If they live by the Great Lakes, there is the high risk for thyroid issues, difficulty with reading, infertility and multiple miscarriages.

If they live by the ocean—whether in Florida, New Jersey, South Carolina, or California—I often notice a natural sharpness in their mind and flow in their speech, because the sea itself fuels intelligence.

Of course, intelligence and good health is everywhere but my focus is on the health and intelligence of people -collectively, per region.

Intelligence and good health is our birthright, but too many people are not getting their share of both. And we need to bring balance where there is imbalance.

I rejoice in the projects, inventions, and ideas that flow when genius and intelligence join hands:

- In **Senegal**, the 164-foot African Renaissance Monument rises—a man, a woman, and a child cast in bronze. It is more than sculpture; it is a declaration that family and nationhood endure.
- In **China**, engineers build sky roads, glass walkways, and underwater highways—visions that seemed impossible a century ago.
- **Finland** did something most nations didn't dare- it put selenium back into the soil. That country-wide choice—protecting whole generations by restoring what the land had lost—is practically unique. Selenium is largely protecting their kidneys from dialysis too.
- In **South Africa**, some citizens speak up to 11 languages. Imagine that brain capacity, that elasticity of mind!
- In **Burkina Faso**, blindness was prevented by red palm oil. A whole community kept its sight because mothers and children received a nutrient nature had already prepared.
- In **Japan and Korea**, people still eat seaweed regularly. They have a large population of elderly people who live beyond 100 years old, escaping many of the chronic diseases that plague North America.

Across America but in the U.S. specifically, I look forward to people of every background caring for the land and the foods we share. I hope American families work together to bring back iodine-rich foods, heal the soil, and revive the old recipes that help our bodies and minds grow strong.

We all live on the same land and eat from the same stores; what one community does affect the others. This new awakening — full of patience, strength, and compassion — will help our children and elders be healthier, smarter and wiser and our communities safer.

Everywhere we look, the story repeats: **when people nourish the mind and body, destiny unfolds.**

Our Legacy of Genius

Black Americans carry a proud legacy of greatness—athletics, academics, arts, and most of all, a history of raising strong, intelligent children. *We will not be dismissed!*

I think of my own Uncle Chris, a genius who was part of a small team in Detroit that figured out how to test the function of the airbag —a breakthrough that has saved the lives of millions of drivers around the world. Although Chris Cobb only received a meek monetary award, his genius idea helped shape our world.

You may not see his name on the official lists of Black American inventors, but we owe him a debt of gratitude. He also worked on bridges that people drive across every day—each crossing a silent testimony to his genius. He represents countless men and women whose names history may never record, yet whose brilliance and labor have shaped the world we live in.

I think about my Uncle Jerry Maholmes, who is also from Detroit who saved lives, not with inventions but with courage and care. Genius is not always a patent or a prize; sometimes it is a life preserved, friends and family protected.

Perhaps you are the mother of a genius child. Perhaps you are the father of an intelligent son. Perhaps you are the genius yourself, using your mind for your family, your community, your world.

Greatness, genius, and good health (mental and physical) is not reserved for a few—it is **our birthright.** A birthright meant for every man, woman and child.

Nourishing the Brain for Destiny

But here is the warning: *A mind cannot rise without its nutrients.* The iodine and selenium we needed in the first 1000 days are needed throughout life. Iodine to light the thyroid and spark intelligence.

- Selenium to protect the brain and guard the thyroid.
- Cod liver oil to strengthen the bones and the immune system.
- Red palm oil to preserve sight and longevity.
- Seaweed to supply minerals the land has forgotten.

Without this, intellect is dimmed, vision is blurred, creativity is sabotaged before birth. With these nutrients, the human spirit soars.

Humanity's Great Feats — A Celebration of Black Genius

When the mind is nourished, humanity creates wonders — not only in stone or steel, but in *thought, innovation, healing, exploration, and transformation.* Here are remarkable figures whose brilliance has shaped our world and lifted human possibility:

Dr. Shirley Ann Jackson — A theoretical physicist and trailblazer, she was the first African-American woman to earn a doctorate at MIT. Her research has *directly contributed to technologies like call waiting and caller ID*, devices millions use daily.

James E. West — Co-inventor of the electret microphone, a technology used in *over 90 % of microphones worldwide* — from phones to hearing aids to recording devices — amplifying voices and ideas.

Where you'll find electret microphones

- Smartphones
- Laptops
- Headsets & earbuds
- Hearing aids
- Baby monitors
- Smart speakers
- Recording devices
- Surveillance & communication equipment everywhere

Mark Dean — A visionary engineer who *co-invented the IBM personal computer* and helped develop the first gigahertz-speed microprocessor, laying foundations for the modern computing era.

Dr. Hadiyah-Nicole Green — A medical physicist pioneering **laser-activated nanoparticle cancer therapies**, pushing the frontiers of precision treatment and offering new hope in the fight against disease.

Vivien Thomas — With brilliant technique and relentless determination, he developed groundbreaking surgical methods to save infants born with complex heart defects, despite beginning his scientific journey unpaid and uncredentialed by institutional barriers.

Dr. Warren Washington — A leading climate scientist whose work on *computer climate models* has deepened humanity's understanding of Earth's changing climate and inspired environmental stewardship.

(And many others) — innovators, brilliant scientists and engineers whose work continues to shape technology, medicine, and discovery.

A Legacy Beyond Measure

These minds did not simply invent tools; they *expanded possibility*. They walked paths untraveled, overcame barriers of bias, and showed that genius — wherever it is found — is humanity's greatest common inheritance.

They remind us:

Genius is not just brilliance — it is the courage to imagine the world not as it is, but as it could be.

Their achievements are monuments of intellect — not of stone, but of thought, perseverance, and heart.

A Call to Destiny

Sisters and brothers: The mind is a terrible thing to waste. Deficiency is not our portion. Destiny is. Feed the mind. Guard the vision. Protect the future.

Because when we nourish the body and soul, we move from **deficiency to destiny.** And when vision is restored, people flourish.

CHAPTER 12

THE SOUL OF A NATION

The soul of a nation is not found in borders or buildings.
It lives in the people — in our sisterhood, our brotherhood, our children, and in the quiet decisions we make when no one is watching.

A Story of Honor

One of Captain Ibrahim Traoré's soldiers was once offered a mountain of money to betray his leader. He paused. He was tempted. But he thought:

"If I take this money, I will have wealth… but no honor.

No respect from my wife.

No pride in my children's eyes."

He refused the offer — choosing honor over profit.

Every life is shaped by choices like this.

Those who killed Martin Luther King Jr., or Malcolm X — did they have choices? Or were they spiritually empty and nutritionally starved? A person can stack supplements on a shelf and still make foolish choices — but what about the person who has never known iodine for four generations?

What happens when the mind is underfed, the soul is under-taught, and wisdom is never passed down?

Ignorance grows.

Impulses rule.

Violence rises.

Not from evil — but from starving brains and wounded judgment.

How Lack of Nourishment Appears in a Community

Remember the tragic story of the children who poured boiling water on a friend at a sleepover — not out of hatred, but out of an inability to foresee consequences.

In a flash of rage, a man strikes the mother of his children. If he could see the consequences — prison, broken homes, fatherless children — he would stop. But clarity requires nourishment.

Parents celebrate early readers, math prodigies, and gifted toddlers — and they should. But learning happens in whole communities, not isolated households.

Your calm child befriends one who cannot regulate emotions or consequences. And suddenly you see nutrition is not individual — it is generational and communal.

The American Paradox

America measures success in salaries, skyscrapers, and degrees. We chased wealth but starved the brain.

We built empires but weakened the soul. We advanced technology while abandoning the womb.

Without nourishment we lose:

- **Clarity.** (the ability to see truth without fog—mentally, emotionally, and morally).
- **Patience.** (ability to wait, endure, or remain calm without frustration, especially during delay, difficulty, or uncertainty).
- **Conscience.** (Your moral awareness, Your sense of responsibility. The part of you that feels guilt, remorse, or peace after a decision).
- **Reason.** (The mind's power to see connections, weigh truth, and choose wisely).

and ultimately —

- **Our moral compass.** (A moral compass is the inner direction that keeps a person oriented toward what is right, even when the world pulls them off course).

Cretinism Has Many Hidden Names: a state of defective mental development, associated with bodily deformity or arrested growth, occurring especially in connection with enlargement of the thyroid gland or goitre.

Idiot. Madness. Foolish. Brainless. Reckless. Simple-minded. Insanity. Stupidity. Thoughtless. Illogical. Irrational. Unsound. Irresponsible. Backward. Mental deficiency. Retardment. Insanity of the mind. Bodily distorted. Curled. Disfigured.

These were never merely insults. They described **biological symptoms of an undernourished brain**. This is what this book is all about – a return to genius and the elimination of cretinism.

Many countries openly celebrate the *elimination of cretinism through iodine sufficiency*. America, however, has lived with its legacy for almost 80 years – not one generation but FOUR!

Now multiply those symptoms of cretinism across hundreds of millions of children and adults and the chaos, confusion, and pain shaping American society over the past 78 years come sharply into focus.

This is not a condition confined to Black communities; it is national—woven into classrooms, courtrooms, households, and the very systems meant to safeguard the mind.

Because when the mind is starved, the soul becomes wounded. And when a whole people are starved, a whole nation collapses from within. We are a nation experiencing a disturbing and preventable deficiency crisis, disguised as:

a behavioral crisis,

a crime crisis,

a mental-health crisis.

THE SOUL OF BLACK AMERICA

What Happened to the Black Culture? An African brother recently asked on social media:

"What is Black culture?"

"What binds Black Americans together?"

"What do Black people stand for?"

He was not being cruel — he was naming a wound he could not see. Because what most of us never knew is that something catastrophic happened to Black America, not only spiritually, emotionally, or socially... but **biologically**.

The longest human experiment in modern history — hidden in plain sight.

Tuskegee: A Known Wound

The Tuskegee Study of untreated syphilis in Black men lasted from **1932 to 1972**. Though the experiment targeted Black men, the pain traveled through entire families. Infected husbands unknowingly passed syphilis to their wives; mothers passed it to their unborn babies. Nineteen infants were born with congenital syphilis, sentenced to lifelong suffering before they took their first breath. And here is the darkest truth:

Penicillin — the cure — became widely available in **1948**, yet it was deliberately withheld. For **twenty-four more years**, Black men, women, and babies were sacrificed so the government could "observe the natural course of the disease."

This was not a medical failure.

This was a *generational betrayal.*

On **May 16, 1997**, President Bill Clinton issued a formal public apology on behalf of the U.S. government.

The Tuskegee Syphilis Study Was A Terrible Atrocity —But It Would Not Be The Last

As the nation reckoned with the legacy of Tuskegee, a far larger public-health crisis was already underway—one that did not affect hundreds, but hundreds of millions across generations! Its reach extended into every womb, every classroom, every neighborhood, and across generations.

The scale of this betrayal was so immense that it altered the trajectory of a people and reshaped the cognitive landscape of the nation.

While America apologized for withholding penicillin in 1948, **that very same year**, another life-saving protection was withheld: the national iodized salt mandate — the single most important public-health tool for preventing cognitive impairment.

A deficiency so severe,

so widespread,

so biologically disruptive,

it altered **collective consciousness** — something never before witnessed in human history.

A nation cannot thrive when its most essential nutrient is missing.

For 78 years, Americans lived without the basic mineral protection nearly every other developed nation adopted.

For 78 years, mothers carried babies without the iodine required to build their brains.

For 78 years, families unknowingly passed deficiency from one generation to the next.

And once you see the pattern—Tuskegee families in clinics, iodine withheld in kitchens—you realize something devastating and heartbreaking:

History repeated itself, but on a scale never seen before in history.

The media captured Black people symptoms but never our sabotage. They were quick to magnify stereotypes: Black on Black crime. High Black incarceration rates, high rates of single motherhood, fatherless homes, broken relationships, broken people, mental dysfunction, and family dysfunction.

They turned our wounds into *headlines.*
They turned our struggles into *entertainment.*
They turned our pain into *profit.*
But they never asked the real questions:

- What weakens a people known for brilliance and spiritual strength?
- What disrupts judgment?
- What erodes impulse control?
- What destabilizes mood, decision-making, and emotional regulation?

They reported the crime —
but never the chronic nutritional collapse behind it.
They condemned the behaviors —
but never the biological sabotage producing them.
Because if America ever told the truth, the whole narrative would collapse:
A population cannot be blamed for symptoms created by state-level neglect and 78 years of iodine starvation.
This was not coincidence.
This was not "Black dysfunction."
This was not cultural failure.
This was **policy-driven biological SABOTAGE** masquerading as personal and communal failure.
And once you see it —
you can never unsee it.

A Study Without Consent

There was no sign-up sheet.
No warnings.
No follow-up.
And yet everyone participated.
The Tuskegee Study involved **600 men.**
The iodine deficiency crisis involved an entire nation across generations!

A deficiency so *powerful* it reshaped IQ, judgment, fertility, child development, thyroid health, immune function, emotional regulation, reading ability, and even collective behavior.

It touched every household.

It infiltrated every generation.

It rewired the biology of a people.

No one consented.

No one was informed.

And every generation paid the price.

The Path Back Home

Now imagine a nation nourished for the past 78 years—
not only with food, but with intention:
iodine, vitamin A, cod liver oil, seaweed, iron —
nutrients for both the body and the mind.
Imagine wisdom passed down at the dinner table,
respect practiced in daily life,
humility carried through the storms.

This is what a soul-fed society looks like

No community escapes the consequences of a nation that starves the mind.

But the path back home remains.

The sea still calls our names.

The foods of our ancestors — iodine, cod liver oil, seaweed — still hold power.

This is a call — not just for supplements, but for soul nourishment: For wisdom passed down. For love lived out. For choices made with clarity and compassion.

Because the soul of a nation is the sum of its people's decisions. And every decision begins in the mind

CHAPTER 13

THE CALL TO ACTION

Sisters—hear me.
1948 was not just a policy failure. It was a generational assault.

A federal iodization bill died, and with it died the protection meant for us. And we have been the ones carrying the cost: pregnancies lost before names were chosen; infants struggling before they learned to crawl; brilliance stolen in the womb before it ever felt the sun; futures redirected into courts and cages instead of classrooms and careers.

Our wombs became battlegrounds. We became the daughters of survivors—surviving hospitals that dismissed our pain, schools that misread our children, and a medical system that never told us the truth.

I write to Black sisters first because the policy assault weighed on us disproportionately and heavy. Then, the ignorance was forced on us. But this call is not ours alone. It reaches every sister, every mother, every grandmother whose family has been robbed of health and clarity.

We heal together.
We rise together.
We refuse to let another generation be stolen.

Our sacred alignment in this lifetime is to midwife a genius nation. Healing moves through us.

In the Book of Genesis, darkness covered the earth, but gross darkness covered the people. For over seventy-eight years, we have lived under that gross darkness—the darkness of not knowing. The darkness of deficiency. The darkness of what was taken from us in silence.

But family—Black America—we will write a new Genesis.

A beginning born in the hands of mothers, fathers, family members, neighbors, friends and children who refuse to accept quietly what was stolen.

We will vacation by the ocean and seas.

We will return to the waters that remember us.

We will buy iodized salt backed by real iodized salt programs even if the salt comes from another country—We will take our iodine, selenium, and red palm oil.

Let our spiritual communities rise and stand in the gap again—just as our ancestors protected the village.

Let our hearts become the storehouse, ensuring every family has iodine salt, selenium and red palm oil.

We can erase mental health crises at the shoreline—the ocean is free! We can rebuild a nation of readers, thinkers, builders, engineers, scientists, and healers—children raised to value family first because **we are family.**

We are who we've been waiting for. This is the moment we remember the firmament is within us—

that the cosmic recipe for health and brilliance was written into our design from the beginning.

We will reclaim our collective memory that was stolen.

We will take back our mental health, our intellect, and our moral clarity. We will reestablish ourselves and strengthen our global bonds only with those who have our highest and best interest at heart.

And in solidarity, we take our place. May every community across the globe honor our journey and uphold our right to health, dignity, and restoration. It starts by not sending your poisonous ingredients to our stores and homes.

To My Black, Melanated, Copper-skinned, Chosen Brothers and Sisters –

What was hidden, withheld, gatekept – is being returned!

The Divine Cosmic Recipe belongs not to governments or rulers, but to every soul, every man, woman, and child.

CHAPTER 14

A NATION'S IODIZED-SALT PROGRAM

Iodized salt protected inland populations. Scandinavia and the Nordic region relied on cod liver oil, with Norway as a leading model. Africa combined both strategies; Asia turned to seaweed; and India, like many nations, relied on iodized salt.

But protecting the intelligence of a nation is never the responsibility of one ministry or one department, it requires a coordinated system *dedicated* to safeguarding every mind.

When even one link breaks, the whole nation slips backward into preventable learning disabilities -backwards in gross darkness, ignorance, special needs and learning disabilities. When the chain is strong, intelligence rises across generations and genius flourishes.

Below is the full architecture of an iodine-salt system.

1. Government & Policy Makers: The Architects of Protection

These leaders decide if the nation protects its children—or leaves them unprotected.

- Ministry of Health
- Ministry of Education
- Ministry of Agriculture
- Food Safety and Standards Authorities
- National Legislators / Parliament
- Customs and Border Control
- Regional and local governments

Their mandate: create mandatory iodization laws, set national standards, enforce compliance, and monitor coverage so every household is protected.

2. Salt Producers & Industry: The Frontline Manufacturers

Salt producers carry one of the most critical responsibilities: adding iodine to the nation's salt supply consistently and correctly.

- Large, medium, and small-scale salt producers
- Artisanal and coastal salt harvesters
- Salt packers and re-packagers
- Salt importers and exporters
- Transport and logistics networks

Their mandate: ensure every grain of salt carries the right amount of iodine from factory to table.

3. Health System & Medical Professionals: The First Responders

These professionals see the impact of iodine deficiency firsthand—in pregnancy loss, thyroid disorders, developmental delays, and learning challenges.

- Physicians (OB/GYNs, pediatricians, endocrinologists)
- Midwives and nurses
- Community health workers
- Hospitals, clinics, and public health institutes
- Medical universities and training programs

Their mandate: educate families, screen mothers and children, detect deficiencies early, and support national campaigns.

4. Education System: The Torchbearers of Knowledge

In many countries, children learned about iodized salt in school before their parents ever heard it mentioned.

- Ministries of Education
- Teachers and school administrators
- Parent–teacher associations
- Universities and research institutions

Their mandate: teach students the truth about iodine and send that knowledge home to families.

5. Families & Communities: The Final Decision-Makers

Even the best national program fails if families do not choose iodized salt.

- Mothers, fathers, grandparents
- Pregnant and breastfeeding women
- Infants, children, and adolescents
- Community leaders
- Churches, mosques, temples, and faith-based groups
- Local NGOs and parent coalitions

Their mandate: buy iodized salt, store it properly, use it daily, and *demand protection* for their children.

6. Retail & Market System: The Gatekeepers

These are the businesses people rely on every day—where iodine protection is either preserved or broken.

- Supermarkets and grocery stores
- Open markets, corner shops, and kiosks
- Wholesale distributors
- Online retailers
- Street vendors

Their mandate: stock adequately iodized salt and remove non-iodized salt from circulation where law requires.

7. Laboratories, Testing, & Monitoring Agencies: The Guardians of Quality

Without monitoring, iodized salt quickly becomes a theory instead of a guarantee.

- National and regional food-testing laboratories
- School and household salt-testing programs

A NATION'S IODIZED-SALT PROGRAM

- Independent quality-control agencies
- Field inspectors and survey teams

Their mandate: measure iodine levels in salt, monitor household coverage, and ensure the nation stays protected.

8. International & Global Partners: The Technical Backbone

No nation builds an iodine program alone. Global support strengthens national capacity.

- World Health Organization (WHO)
- United Nations International Children's Emergency Fund (UNICEF)
- Iodine Global Network (IGN)
- Global Alliance for Improved Nutrition (GAIN)
- World Bank and philanthropic foundations

Their mandate: provide global guidance, training, data, and technical support so nations can maintain universal salt iodization.

9. Media & Communication Networks: The Voice of the Nation

Public understanding determines the success of any health program.

- National radio and television
- Newspapers and journalists
- Social-media educators and influencers
- Public-health campaign designers
- Faith radio, community radio, and local messengers

Their mandate: make iodine a household word—simple, urgent, and unavoidable!

Note: A mandate is an official order or requirement that must be followed. It is stronger than a suggestion—it means something is mandatory, required by law, or required by an authority. It is not voluntary either.

Why All These Stakeholders Matter

*Iodine protection is national intelligence protection.
*It is maternal health protection.

It is the future protection.

One weak link—one region left behind, one factory cutting corners, one doctor untrained, one school uninformed—can steal potential from a whole generation.

But when every stakeholder does their part, a nation sees:

- *higher literacy*
- *fewer miscarriages*
- *stronger cognitive outcomes*
- *healthier pregnancies*
- *smarter, more capable children ready to learn*
- *a more prepared, more intelligent future workforce*
- *generational intelligence*

Iodized salt is the smallest intervention with the largest return on a nation's intelligence.

The **Genius Revolution** is not merely an ending—

it is a beginning, a return, a remembering.

A spiritual rebirth of a people awakening to their collective brilliance.

A rising of minds, of families, of the Black community who finally remember who they are- The Chosen Ones.

Stand tall.

Vote with vision.

Demand with courage.

Manifest with divine authority.

We are fragments of **Divine Intelligence**, wrapped in flesh, walking the earth with purpose. And now, together, we rise.

We rise in our genius.

We rise to greatness.

We rise in our truth.

We rise in power.

We rise as one great impregnable (*unstoppable*) people. Remember, we are who we've been waiting for.

CHAPTER 15

THE CASE FOR PUBLIC HEALTH REPARATIONS

For over seventy-eight years, the United States allowed a preventable nutritional deficiency to quietly sabotage the cognitive potential of well over 1/2 billion children and adults – across timelines and generations.

Iodine deficiency—long recognized by global scientists as the leading cause of preventable brain damage—was permitted to persist in a nation with every resource, every technology, and every opportunity to eliminate it.

My son was one of those harmed

He was born into a country that had the knowledge to protect his developing brain yet chose not to act on that knowledge. His severe learning disability is not an isolated medical event—it is part of a national pattern. He is one story among millions of children who are now adults and whose potential was shaped, limited, or lost because of a deficiency that should never have existed!

This is not just a personal loss. It is a generational betrayal.

A Public Health Failure on a National Scale

A government has a sacred duty to safeguard public health. That duty does not dissolve simply because the harm is nutritional instead of chemical or developmental instead of sudden.

When a nation knows how to prevent a condition, when the tools are available, when the science is overwhelmingly clear—*inaction becomes a form of negligence and genocide. And 78-plus years of inaction becomes generations under attack!*

For decades, the failure to ensure adequate iodine intake—especially for pregnant women, infants, and growing children—created a silent epidemic that would ripple throughout the world!

These outcomes were not surprising; they were predicted! For almost a century, scientific literature has warned that insufficient iodine during pregnancy results in irreversible neurological impairment across the spectrum.

And yet, for seventy-eight (78) plus years, the United States allowed this to continue.

Why Reparations Must Be Considered

When preventable harm stretches across generations, the question of accountability becomes unavoidable. Reparations are not about punishment. They are about **acknowledgment, responsibility, and repair.**

Reparations answer three moral questions:

1. **Was harm done?**
   Yes. Millions of children, women and adults suffered cognitive injury, thyroid issues, and generational devestation that was entirely preventable.
2. **Was the harm avoidable?**
   Yes. The science was clear, and the tools existed.
3. **Did inaction contribute to the harm?**
   Yes. Regulatory failure allowed iodine deficiency to persist unchecked for multiple generations.

When these truths converge, reparations become not only reasonable—**they become a matter of justice.**

What Public Health Reparations Would Look Like

Payouts for my son and me; payouts for families and repair for the nation. Reparations are not a check—they are a blueprint for healing.

Public health reparations should include

1. *Mandatory Universal Iodine Fortification*
   A nationwide initiative ensuring that every family receives the protection they were denied.
2. *Support for Affected Children and Adults*

Funding for cognitive therapies, educational interventions, job training, and lifelong support.

3. *Real Maternal and Infant Nutrition Programs*
Targeted investments in prenatal care, iodine, red palm oil, and selenium supplementation, and national public-health education.

4. *Formal Acknowledgment and Public Apology*
Recognition for the millions harmed by a failure that should never have occurred. Reparations are not a political gesture. They are restoration. They are the bridge between historic harm and a healthier, more equitable future.

My Family's Story as Evidence of a National Issue

I share my son's story not to evoke pity, but to reveal the cost of inaction—the potential he carried but could not fully access because his nation failed to protect his developing brain.

His struggled in school—his processing challenges, his lifelong learning disability—were not destiny. They were the outcome of a preventable deficiency. And though I celebrate his brilliance, his gifts, and every way he continues to rise, I also carry the truth: this never had to be his battle – our battle.

My story is personal, but it is not unique. And that is precisely the tragedy. Millions of families across the nation have a similar story hidden in different words, tucked inside IEP meetings, doctor visits, behavior charts, prisons, death, quiet heartbreak, and lifelong pain.

A Call for Federal Responsibility

A government that fails to act on established science fails its people. The United States had the knowledge, the resources, and a fully capable public-health infrastructure to eliminate iodine deficiency. Yet for four generations, it did not – (*not one, two or three but 4 generations that continues to suffer*).

It is not radical to demand accountability.

It is not extreme to seek restoration.

It is not unreasonable to say: **Make this right!**

Reparations represent more than financial justice.

They represent moral clarity. This chapter is not only about what happened. It is about what the nation must choose to do next:

- acknowledge the truth,
- repair the harm,
- and ensure that no future child is born into a preventable cognitive deficit.

This is how we honor what was stolen—and how we spark a Genius Revolution for generations to come.

Global Iodine Deficiency Day — October 21

The Day the World Remembers the Mineral That Protects the Mind and Prevents Learning Disabilities

Every year on **October 21**, countries around the world pause to recognize one truth:

Iodine deficiency is the leading cause of preventable intellectual disability on earth

This day is known as **Global Iodine Deficiency Day** (also called *Global IDD Day*), established in **1992** by the World Health Organization (WHO), UNICEF, and the Iodine Global Network. It is not a holiday — it is a global alarm clock ringing once a year to remind nations:

Protect your mothers.
Protect your children.
Protect the future.

Why October 21 Matters

On this day, *governments, ministries of health, schools, and public-health leaders* unite across continents to:

- Raise awareness about the dangers of iodine deficiency
- Promote iodized salt as a universal protection
- Educate mothers and families about iodine's role in pregnancy and early brain development
- Celebrate progress in nations that eliminated iodine deficiency
- Call attention to places that are still at risk

Some countries hold parades, school campaigns, billboards, radio messages, and community events. In several nations — like Kazakhstan, China, Ethiopia, and parts of Latin America — children learn about iodine in school the same way American children learn about fire safety or brushing their teeth. (*How insulting is this*)?

A Global Celebration

While the world was educating its families, fortifying its salt, and preventing *millions* of cases of intellectual disability, most Americans never heard a word about Global IDD Day.

- No national campaign
- No school education
- No public-health messaging
- No reminders for mothers
- No awareness for fathers

For over **three decades**, the world has been celebrating a program designed to **protect the next generation's intelligence**, while the United States and their institutions remained silent.

The Purpose of Global IDD Day

The mission is simple, powerful, and universal:
To prevent a child from losing 10–15 IQ points before they are even born.
When a nation embraces iodine, literacy rises, productivity increases, and the collective intellect strengthens.

What Global IDD Day Represents

It represents the world's commitment to never again allow a generation to suffer from preventable cognitive harm.

It represents:

- **education** over ignorance
- **prevention** over suffering
- **nutrition** over disease labels
- **protection** over negligence

It represents the belief that every child — no matter their nation — deserves a nourished brain. *They deserve the opportunity to fulfil their highest human potential!*

Rise and Shine

Take your selenium & iodine
and let the glory of
Divine Intelligence
be seen on us!

SECTION 2

GENERATIONAL HEALTH & LONGEVITY

Chapters 16 – 34

CHAPTER 16

BREAD – ONCE A SYMBOL OF LIFE

Bread has always been a symbol of life.

"Give us this day our daily bread," we pray.

But in America, bread is no longer life-giving—it is toxic. The very food meant to nourish families has been laced with chemicals that poison the body, weaken the thyroid, and fuel the epidemic of cancer that is destroying our communities.

America's Daily Bread – A Poisoned Loaf

Here in the U.S., **bromated flour** is still on the shelves— baked into breads, buns, bagels, biscuits, muffins, noodles and pizza dough. Every bite risks exposure to a **carcinogen**.

The ingredient labels are often clear! Listed on the package is the poison used to destroy us! Toddlers eat it, children eat at home and school, and adults eat it, usually every day.

Think about it: The price of bread is not $6.99 anymore. The true cost for bread and bake goods in the U.S. is a **heart**, a **kidney**, a **liver**, a **pancreas**, a **life**. Souls are far too high a price for our bread.

The Bromide Dominance Theory

Scientists have given a name to what we're witnessing: The Bromide Dominance Theory.

When iodine is missing from the body, other halides—like *fluoride, chlorine, and bromine*—move in and take its place. These imposters act like squatters in the cells, blocking iodine and disrupting everything that keeps the body alive and clear-minded. Instead of life, they bring slow death:

- Cancer of the breast, thyroid, ovary, and prostate.

- Skin disorders: rashes, eczema, and severe acne.
- Psychological distress: paranoia, fatigue, depression.
- Cardiac arrhythmia—when the heart beats out of rhythm, too fast or too slow.
- Neurological decline—when the brain and nerves begin to weaken, making it harder to think, remember, or move as you once did.

Examples of Neurological Decline

1. Cognitive and Mental Changes

    - *Memory loss* (short-term or long-term)
    - *Difficulty concentrating* or focusing
    - *Slow thinking* or decision-making
    - *Poor judgment* or loss of reasoning ability (making choices that don't make sense).
    - *Confusion or disorientation*
    - *Reduced problem-solving skills or creativity*

2. Emotional and Behavioral Changes

    - Irritability, aggression, or sudden mood swings
    - Anxiety, depression, or apathy (loss of motivation)
    - Loss of empathy or emotional flatness (when a person stops showing feelings or has trouble caring about others' emotions). They may seem distant, cold, or disconnected
    - Social withdrawal or loss of interest in previously enjoyed activities

3. Physical and Motor Symptoms

    - *Tremors* or shaking hands
    - *Muscle weakness* or stiffness
    - *Poor coordination or balance* (frequent falls)
    - *Slowed movement* (bradykinesia)
    - *Difficulty walking* or dragging one foot
    - *Speech changes* (slurred words, slower speech

4. Sensory and Perceptual Problems

- Blurred or double vision
- Loss of smell or taste
- Tingling, numbness, or burning sensations (neuropathy)
- Heightened or dull response to touch or pain

5. Systemic Issues

- *Irregular heartbeat or blood pressure* (linked to brainstem dysfunction)
- *Sleep disturbances* (insomnia, vivid dreams, or sleep paralysis)
- *Digestive problems* (constipation or loss of appetite)

One last system issue is temperature regulation problems — feeling cold even in extreme heat

Iodine deficiency can weaken the thyroid so much that the body struggles to regulate temperature. The thyroid sets your *metabolic thermostat*. When it doesn't have enough iodine, that thermostat turns down too low.

This means:

- Your body produces less heat.
- Your circulation slows.
- Your cells burn less energy.

So even if the temperature outside is hot — **your internal temperature is cold** because your thyroid cannot produce enough hormones to warm the body from the inside out.

This is why someone with iodine deficiency may sit in the sun and still feel chilled to the bone or enter a warm room and still need a sweater. It's not "in their head." It's biology.

When iodine is restored, the thyroid wakes back up, metabolism increases, and the body's thermal engine begins to regulate properly again.

This is why bromate is not banned in our breads, flours, and everyday flour by-products—because in an iodine-deficient nation, chaos follows both inside the body and out.

When the body lacks iodine, its natural defender, the invader wins. And when iodine disappears from the table, confusion appears in the home, in the classroom, and in the nation.

You see the pattern.

Without iodine, everything falls apart!

Potassium bromate destroys our organs, especially the kidneys

So let us ask the only question that matters:

- Who added potassium bromate to our bread?
- Who approved it?
- And who still allows it to poison millions?

The moment poison entered the recipe, we stopped being "patients with compromised kidney issues." We became **victims** of a system that sanctioned harm.

- **Patient** — a neutral term, someone receiving medical care.
- **Victim** — someone harmed by an action, a system, a crime.

Once poison is knowingly administered, illness is no longer "natural." It is engineered.

One person poisoned is murder.

Three people poisoned is mass murder.

But when **millions** are poisoned? That is not a public-health concern, but **genocide by design.**

And the tragedy is this:

Had iodine never been removed from the flour, bromine could never have taken its place.

Bromate only dominates when the body is starved of iodine — the very mineral that shields the kidneys, brain, and immune system.

Now, the truth can no longer be ignored.

Where Bromate is Banned

- European Union – banned in all foods.
- Canada – delisted in **1994**. That was **30 years ago!**
- China – banned since **2005**. That was **20 years ago!**
- Brazil – banned in **1998**. That was **27 years ago!**

These countries recognized the risk and responded. They chose food, not poisons. They chose children's futures, not corporate margins. They chose life over death.

Where It's Not Banned

United States.

The FDA still allows potassium bromate in specific flours—up to **50 ppm** in bromated flour and **75 ppm** in bromated whole-wheat flour. (*Higher in whole wheat*).

It must appear on the label—but most people never notice.

United States.

California's Food Safety Act (AB 418)—signed October 7, 2023—bans potassium bromate (along with Red Dye 3, brominated vegetable oil, and propylparaben) in foods sold in the state beginning **January 1, 2027**.

Genocide in America

Crime scene location - America - operates like a crime scene. Every crime has a motive, a weapon, perpetrators, accomplices, and victims.

The motive? Profit and control.

The weapons? Everyday poisonous foods and policies.

The victims? Americans -Black, Hispanic, Pacific Islanders, Whites and then everyone within reach.

Industrial additives, dyes, and contaminants are widespread in our food system; examples include potassium bromate, aspartame, perchlorates, mercury, lead, cadmium, fluoride, titanium dioxide, glyphosate, propylene glycol and more. These are not "accidents"; they are tolerated exposures with foreseeable harm.

The human body is delicate. Our organs, tissues, and cells are all delicate and cannot manage the everyday stress of poisons. One poison alone is killing us; What it doesn't do, the other poisons will. Disease? Murder? Mass murder? It's all the same.

Call it what it is - GENOCIDE!

If the outcome is mass disability, shortened lives, and erased potential—especially along racial and economic lines—what else should we call it?

- For Black Americans, it's about removal from native land and erasure of our ancient wisdom, stolen inheritance, and premature demise.
- For everyone else who lives in America - it's collateral—proximity poisoning.

These Numbers Are Not Diseases, But Evidence and Proof of Harm

- **35.5 million** Americans live with kidney disease.
- **815,000** live with kidney failure.
- **555,000** are on dialysis.

Risk of Kidney Failure vs. White Americans:

- Black Americans (Indigenous): **4× higher**
- Hispanic Americans: **2× higher**
- Native Americans: **2× higher**
- Asian Americans: **1.4× higher**

Slow deaths, premature loss and graves everywhere—while the perpetrators walk free.

No One Held to Account

California took a step—banning several additives (including potassium bromate) **beginning in 2027**—but tomorrow's promise won't resurrect yesterday's losses and today's tragedy.

Meanwhile, policy makers and their donors- food conglomerates, chemical suppliers, medical institutions, and the sliver of the 1% that profits—escape accountability.

A Silent War While America Sleeps

A slow violence. We don't die on the same day; we die on the same timeline—not suddenly, not loud. Slow. Synchronized. We keep focusing on the damage (kidney disease, dialysis, kidney failure, cancers, etc.) while the murderers and their accomplices get away.

A damaged brain can't rally; a confused mind can't organize; broken bodies can't march or advocate.

The Verdict & The Mandate

It's transparency time. Ban bromate. Feed truth. Restore iodine and selenium where they belong—in policy, in food, in prenatal care, in daily life.

Because a nation that starves its people of health starves its own genius.

CHAPTER 16 BIBIOGRAPHY

1. **International Agency for Research on Cancer (IARC).** *Potassium Bromate. IARC Monographs on the Evaluation of Carcinogenic Risks to Humans*, vol. 73. Lyon: International Agency for Research on Cancer, 1999.
   (Classified as Group 2B: Possible human carcinogen.)

2. **Kurokawa, Y., A. Maekawa, M. Takahashi, and Y. Hayashi.** "Toxicity and Carcinogenicity of Potassium Bromate—A New Renal Carcinogen." *Environmental Health Perspectives* 87 (1990): 309–335.
   (Renal and thyroid tumors in rats.)

3. **Ballmaier, D., and B. Epe.** "DNA Damage by Bromate: Mechanism and Consequences." *Toxicology* 221, nos. 2–3 (2006): 166–171.
   (Oxidative DNA damage; mutagenicity.)

4. **Entezam, A., et al.** "Potassium Bromate: A Potent DNA-Oxidizing Agent." *DNA Repair* (2010).
   (PMC review article summarizing mechanistic toxicology.)

5. **De Vriese, A., R. Vanholder, and N. Lameire.** "Severe Acute Renal Failure Due to Bromate Intoxication." *Nephrology Dialysis Transplantation* 12, no. 1 (1997): 204–209.
   (Human poisoning: gastrointestinal irritation leading to acute kidney injury.)

6. **Hamada, F., et al.** "A Case of Acute Potassium Bromate Intoxication." *Japanese Journal of Toxicology* (1990).
   (Documented vomiting, diarrhea, abdominal pain, and anuric renal failure.)

7. **Elsheikh, A. S., et al.** "Effects of Potassium Bromate on Male Rat Growth and Testicular Histology." *Journal of Taibah University for Science* 10, no. 4 (2016): 543–555.
   (Reproductive toxicity; reduced testicular and epididymal metrics.)

8. **Nwonuma, C. O., et al.** "Testicular Toxicity in Rats Administered Potassium Bromate: Histopathological and Biochemical Evidence." *Journal of Taibah University for Science* 10, no. 4 (2016): 520–528.

9. **Food Safety and Standards Authority of India (FSSAI).** *Final List of Food Additives: Ban on Potassium Bromate in Foods.* New Delhi: FSSAI, 2016.
   (Policy action; similar bans exist in the EU, UK, Canada, Brazil, Nigeria, and others.)

CHAPTER 17

EXPERIMENT ON RATS, NOT GOD'S PEOPLE

In science, animals and rodents are often used to test what food, chemicals, and drugs will do to the human body. But what happens when the same harmful experiments are conducted on God's people without their knowledge?

The Rat Experiment

There was an experiment with three groups of rats:

Group One was fed nourishing food. The rats grew to normal size, remained calm, gentle, social and could be handled without fear of being bitten.

Group Two received less nourishment. They were smaller, but still friendly and non-aggressive.

Group Three starved of proper nutrients, showed the most dramatic change. These rats became overweight, constipated, hostile, and quick to attack. Their temperament shifted toward violence—against each other and against the researchers.

The difference? **The state of their brains.**

Malnourishment damaged their mental stability, creating aggression, confusion, and dysfunction from the inside out.

Now pause and consider: How different are our communities today?

How many children, teens, and adults are reacting in aggression and violence not because they are "bad," but because their brains—like those rats—are starving. Starving for minerals. Starving for iodine. Starving for nutrients their minds were never given!

What we call "misbehavior" is often simply malnourished brains trying to survive.

The Aspartame Crisis – The Biological War Continues

Fast forward to today. A chemical called **aspartame**—sold under names like *NutraSweet, Equal, Sugar Twin, and Ajinomoto*—is added to over **2,500 products in the United States** [U.S. FDA, 2021]. From diet sodas to "sugar-free" candies, it is marketed as *safe*, even *"healthy."* Sadly, these sugar packages sit right on the tables of the restaurants we frequent.

But here is the truth:

- In the United States, **pregnant women** are among the highest consumers of aspartame-containing soft drinks—often to avoid weight gain during pregnancy [Humphries, Pretorius & Naudé, 2008].
- That means their **babies are exposed in the womb.**
- Research has linked fetal aspartame exposure to an increased risk of **leukemia and other cancers in children** [Soffritti et al., 2007; Schernhammer et al., 2012].

Here's the clue: when you see the word **"Zero"** on a label—like *"Zero Sugar," "Zero Soda," or "Zero Calories"*—that is a red flag. Most of the time, it means the product has been sweetened with aspartame or another artificial chemical substitute. What looks like "zero" is really *poison hiding in plain sight*.

The Real Rat Experiment

Aspartame: The Zero That Costs Us Everything. Before aspartame ever reached store shelves, the lab animals told the truth. Rats fed aspartame **died again and again** during safety testing. The trials failed. The evidence was clear.

But the chemical was pushed through anyway — approved not because it was safe, but because the industry insisted it must be sold.

Rats don't buy "Zero" sodas from school vending machines either, but our children do. They drink them daily, sometimes all day, sitting in classrooms where their brains are still forming — while the chemical inside those bottles have been linked to tumors, neurological damage, and developmental delays.

Now look around: Classrooms filled with children who can't sit still, can't focus, can't speak clearly, or struggle to learn.

Teens wrestling with anxiety, rage, panic attacks, and depression. Adults showing unprecedented rates of cancer, diabetes, memory loss, and neurological disorders — conditions once considered rare.

Meanwhile, the food system continues to sell us chemicals never meant for human consumption, wrapped in bright labels and empty promises. "Zero sugar" ... "Zero calories" ... but the real cost is hidden.

When you see 'Zero' on the bottle, treat it as a warning — not an achievement.
Zero nourishment.
Zero safety.
Zero benefit.
Zero protection.

And the payback is unfolding in real time, in our homes, our schools, and our communities.

Europe Moves While America Sleeps

A petition has already called for aspartame to be banned in 11 European countries—including Germany, France, Spain, Italy, Ireland, and the United Kingdom [NutraIngredients, 2023]. These nations recognize the danger and are moving to protect their people.

Meanwhile, in America, aspartame remains in thousands of products—quietly consumed daily by children, pregnant women, and families.

God's Plan vs. Man's Experiment

Divine Intelligence never intended for us to be test subjects, but capitalism clearly does. Instead of nourishment, we are sold dyes, preservatives, artificial sweeteners, toxic chemicals and poisons.

Instead of brilliance, our minds were dulled. Instead of peace, we inherited aggression, dysfunction, disease, early decline and death.

The lesson from the rat experiments are clear: malnourished brains breed chaos. The lesson from aspartame is even clearer: chemicals do not belong in our children, our wombs, or our communities.

Bottom Line

When you see the word *Zero*, don't be fooled. It may not mean "nothing"—it may mean **aspartame.** Protect yourself. Protect your children.

Nourish your brain with the foods of creation, not the chemicals of industry. Because once the brain is damaged, the soul struggles to fulfill its divine purpose.

Aspartame: Where It Hides

- **Zero** Sugar Sodas
- Diet Drinks
- Sugar-Free Gum
- "Light" Yogurts
- Protein Shakes & Bars
- Flavored Waters
- Candies & Desserts

2. **Health Risks**

   - *Brain Fog & Mood Swings*
   - *Headaches & Seizures*
   - *Aggression & Anxiety*
   - *Cancer Risk (linked in studies)*
   - *Fertility Issues*
   - *Childhood Leukemia Risk*

3. **Who's at Risk Most**

   Children
   Pregnant Women
   Seniors

4. **God's Foods for Sweetness**

   - Raw Honey
   - Fruit
   - Dates

   The health of the mother is the health of the generation.

CHAPTER 17 BIBLIOGRAPHY

1. **Soffritti, M., et al.** "Aspartame Induces Lymphomas and Leukemias in Rats." *Environmental Health Perspectives* 115, no. 9 (2007): 1293–1297.
2. **Schernhammer, E. S., et al.** "Consumption of Artificial Sweetener- and Sugar-Containing Soda and Risk of Lymphoma and Leukemia in Men and Women." *American Journal of Clinical Nutrition* 96, no. 6 (2012): 1419–1428.
3. **Humphries, P., E. Pretorius, and H. Naudé.** "Direct and Indirect Cellular Effects of Aspartame on the Brain." *European Journal of Clinical Nutrition* 62, no. 4 (2008): 451–462.
4. **U.S. Food and Drug Administration.** *Additional Information about High-Intensity Sweeteners Permitted for Use in Food*. Silver Spring, MD: FDA, 2021.
5. **NutraIngredients.** "Petition to Ban Aspartame in the EU Gains Traction." *NutraIngredients.com*, 2023.

CHAPTER 18

HESITATE BEFORE YOU CELEBRATE

I am convinced the people of the United States have been manipulated into celebrating their own sickness, their own suffering, and their own premature deaths. We clap, we wear ribbons, we march and we chant—but very few stop to ask: *Why are we celebrating conditions that were preventable in the first place?*

Before women can protect their children, we must learn to heal and protect ourselves. Sisters, if you understood the full depth of the forces working against our families, you would hesitate before ever joining these "celebrations." These patriarchal institutions have trained us—cunningly—to participate in our own destruction.

They play a deadly game of good cop/bad cop with our lives:

- One institution poisons our bread, water, and food with chemicals that cause disease.
- Another institution pretends to save us by cutting, burning, or drugging the symptoms.
- One creates the disease.
- The other sells itself as the cure.

And in the middle of this manipulation, the people suffer. Women get sick. Children break down. Families crumble. All while being told to "celebrate awareness" instead of demanding prevention.

Revelation Unfolding

In *Revelation 12:4*, it reads

"The dragon stood before the woman who was ready to give birth, to devour her child as soon as it was born."

Who is the dragon today?

And how do we recognize evil in our time?

You don't need fire-breathing monsters or horns to identify danger. Start by watching the systems that withhold micronutrients from men, women and children.

Watch the institutions that leave mothers iodine-deficient, babies vulnerable, and families confused.

Watch the ones that deny you the minerals God placed in creation for your protection.

And pay close attention to the voices that invite you—subtly, beautifully, convincingly—

to **celebrate your own sickness**,

your own decline,

your own premature death.

Evil today is not always loud;

sometimes it smiles, hands you a ribbon,

and asks you to march.

But wisdom recognizes the dragon by its fruits:

Be cautious of anything that harms the mind, weakens the womb, steals the children, or convinces a nation to applaud its own destruction.

Why Are We Celebrating?

- We celebrate **"Disabilities Awareness Week"** when iodine deficiency is the single leading cause of intellectual disabilities and physical disabilities. Mothers, you must know: if your child has already been injured, even from something as devastating as vaccines, you still have the power to detoxify and nourish their brain with minerals. Healing is not gone—it is waiting for you to claim it.

Disabilities are not *what happened* to our children, it is the harm that *was done* to our children.

- We celebrate **"Deaf and Blind Awareness Month"** as if hearing loss and vision loss are inevitable. But they are not. Hearing decline can be detected early and prevented early, and blindness and vision loss can be prevented entirely—not by a doctor, but by mothers armed with the wisdom of Mother Nature.

We celebrate **"Breast Cancer Awareness Month"** with ribbons and charity walks. But how many of these campaigns teach women to eat foods like seaweed, take iodine and selenium that prevent cancer in the first place?

Where are the commercials advertising seaweed, iodine, selenium, and red palm oil? Where are the banners reminding us that what we eat and what we neglect to eat determines whether cancer has room to grow?

The Truth About Prevention

Mother Nature has always carried the prevention within her. The sea is rich with iodine, minerals, and fucoidan—a powerful compound found in brown seaweeds (wakame, Kombu/kelp, Masuku) that supports the immune system, prevents tumor growth, and protects against degenerative diseases.

Instead of parading in the streets celebrating diseases, we should be in our kitchens reclaiming the remedies that prevent them. We should be at our tables teaching our daughters and sons how to nourish their brains, their thyroids, their hearts, and their eyes.

We should be passing down recipes made with seaweed not passing down stories of diagnoses, fear and surgeries.

Sisters, A Call to Return

Like a remote control to a toy car, our wombs, our health, our children's brain are being manipulated by systems. We must return to wisdom. We must return to the foods of the ocean, the blessings of the earth, and the guidance of Divine Intelligence.

Sisters, hesitate before you celebrate. Ask yourself: *Am I celebrating prevention, or am I celebrating the chains of disease?*

Because true awareness is not in the ribbon—it is in the knowledge that cancer, diabetes, blindness, obesity, Alzheimer's, Parkinson's, and even AIDS are not random punishments from above, but conditions linked to deficiencies that could have been addressed if we had only remembered the ocean's gifts.

Celebration vs. Prevention

What Society Celebrates -

- Disabilities Awareness Week → Passively accepting learning struggles as "normal."

- Deaf and Blind Awareness Month → Passively accepting hearing and vision loss as "fate."
- Breast Cancer Awareness Month → Passively accepting cancer as inevitable and breast mutilation as "the only way to restore health."

What Mothers Can Do Instead

- **Iodine & Selenium** → Support brain development, prevent learning disabilities.
- **Vitamin A & Red Palm Oil** → Protect eyesight, prevent childhood blindness.
- **Fucoidan from seaweed** → Strengthen immunity, prevent tumor growth.
- **Cod Liver Oil & Ocean Foods** → Support thyroid, heart, and whole-body health.

Truth

Awareness without prevention is a trap!

Mother Nature already gave us the wisdom to prevent what America wants us to celebrate. Be mindful and don't celebrate your own demise.

CHAPTER 19

WITHOUT VISION, THE PEOPLE PERISH

A Scripture and a Warning

"Where there is no vision, the people perish." (Proverbs 29:18)

This verse is more than poetry. It is prophecy, biology, and reality. For vision is both **sight of the eyes** and **sight of the mind**. Without either, futures are stolen, destiny cut short, generations left wandering in the dark.

And yet, much of this blindness is preventable. Not fate. Not chance. But preventable malnutrition—especially Vitamin A deficiency, which blinds children worldwide before they reach their fifth birthday.

If vision perishes, so do possibilities.

Blindness: A Global Scandal

Vitamin A deficiency is one of the biggest health problems in the world. When kids don't get enough vitamin A, they may not grow well, can lose their eyesight, and are at risk for infections. Also, Vitamin A deficiency is a risk factor for cognitive impairment and mental illness.

The World Health Organization posits that about 190 million young children and 19 million pregnant women around the world don't get enough vitamin A. That makes vitamin A deficiency one of the top reasons people have serious health problems.

In West Africa, Vitamin A deficiency once left villages filled with children who could not see at dusk. In Asia, entire clinics overflowed with mothers carrying infants whose eyes had already clouded with night blindness.

- In **Burkina Faso**, supplementation with *red palm oil* restored night vision in 90% of deficient children (Zeba et al., 2006).
- In **India**, fortification programs with Vitamin A rich oils reversed epidemic childhood blindness within communities.
- In **Indonesia**, children given *red palm oil* instead of capsules thrived, proving that food-based solutions could save more lives than pills.
- In **Tanzania and Ghana**, families who never abandoned *red palm oil* traditions show some of the lowest rates of night blindness.

Meanwhile, in **the United States**, we are told Vitamin-A deficiency is "rare." But 45–90% of Americans show inadequate Vitamin A intake! How then do we explain the epidemic of glasses, bifocals, cataracts, glaucoma, floaters, macular degeneration, vision loss, blindness and more.

If Vitamin A deficiency blinds a child in Africa, what makes us think it does not weaken the eyes of children in Atlanta, Chicago, or Los Angeles?

The truth: when nations abandon protective foods, blindness and brain fog follows.

The Gatekeepers

Sisters, mothers, grandmothers—you are the gatekeepers. You season the soup. You stir the oatmeal, millet and quinoa. **You choose the oils.**

Just as African mothers ladle *red palm oil* into stews, you too hold the power to shield your children's eyes from darkness. This one food—pressed from the fruit of the palm—carries in its crimson glow the very compounds that *prevent blindness, fuel immunity, and strengthen the brain.*

And let us be clear: blindness is not only of the eyes. There is a blindness of intellect, a blindness of memory, a blindness of spirit. When children are robbed of nutrients in the womb or at the table, they stumble in school, they struggle to focus, they forget how to dream.

But when mothers restore red palm oil to their kitchens, light returns—not just to the eyes, but to the mind.

Children 5 Years Old are at Risk of Vision Loss

Sadly, famous musicians like **Stevie Wonder** lost his eyesight as a 6-month-old baby, and **Ray Charles** lost his vision before he was seven years old. We cannot say for sure if it was because of vitamin A deficiency. But what we do know is that millions of other children around the world have also lost their sight, many without their stories ever being told.

The World Health Organization calls Vitamin A deficiency one of the leading preventable causes of childhood blindness worldwide. But just like iodine, women in America, didn't get this information either. Yet here at home, we have been led to believe it is "not an issue." Meanwhile, glasses become normal at age six, and cataract surgeries routine by age sixty.

But in **West Africa**, elderly people still read without glasses into their 80s and 90s, their vision preserved by diets rich in red palm oil, palm fruit, and local greens.

In **Okinawa, Japan**, where iodine-rich seaweeds and fish oils remain staples, elders maintain sharp vision and sharp minds well past 100 years old.

In **Andean villages of South America**, where native diets once overflowed with carotenoid-rich tubers and greens, blindness was rare—until imported processed foods replaced tradition.

What does this tell us? Where natural foods remain, vision remains. Where food systems are corrupted, sight perishes.

My Testimony

For ten years, I drove my son to the ophthalmologist's office. Ten years of yearly specialized screenings, co-pays, polite handshakes — and no real answers.

Not once did anyone tell me that nutrients like **red palm oil and selenium,** could protect my son's vision. Not once did anyone mention that his eye disorder could be connected to a congenital thyroid issue related to *iodine* deficiency. For a decade, the truth sat in silence.

I thought I was practicing "prevention." But I wasn't.

I was in an **automatic, zombie-like routine** — appointment after appointment, test after test, expecting different results. That's what insanity looks like. Meanwhile, no one could ever explain my son's diagnosis. It took me to begin researching to understand nystagmus and astigmatism could have been preventable.

Blindness, vision loss, imperfect vision are not inevitable with birth or age — they are symptoms of deficiency. We were designed to have strong vision all the days of our life.

My son is now 23. I fight every day to protect his vision. And I carry the weight of what I didn't know: If I had understood iodine, selenium, and red palm oil back then, my son would have perfect vision today.

And I am not alone. There are *millions* in America who went to the doctor faithfully and still went blind — just like there are millions who went to the dentist faithfully and still lost all their teeth.

Because *yearly appointments are not prevention programs.*

Think about it: If your health continues to decline year after year, then there is no prevention — only routine.

True prevention comes from the gifts of nature:

the trees, the seas, the soil, the sun.

There are no prevention programs in the U.S., only appointments. And there is no such thing as disease in remission. How can you have remission without the gifts of the firmament.

Today, I am grateful for the revelation that mothers hold the power to preserve sight. I use red palm oil and selenium for my family's eye health — not just for my son, but for all of us. Even my granddaughter, only ten years old, already wears glasses. And I refuse to accept that glasses at ten are "normal." I refuse to accept that vision loss is "inevitable."

If mothers reclaim this wisdom, sabotage ends here.

Blindness ends here.

Without Vision, People Perish

When a child loses sight, they lose more than eyesight —they lose opportunities, confidence, safety, mental health, and their futures.

When a *people* lose vision, they lose direction, wisdom, and hope. Blindness of the eyes leads to blindness of the mind — and both lead to stolen destinies.

This is another reason why I named this book **Stolen Intellect.**

Because if sight is stolen, if intellect is dulled, then futures are sabotaged before they even begin.

If mothers rise, a nation rises.

If vision returns, intellect returns.

If nourishment is restored, genius awakens.

My Personal Red Palm Oil Testimony

I first came across red palm oil while reading about brain health. Unsure but curious, I tried it. I began adding a spoonful into my bowl of soup and even into hot tea.

What happened surprised me. For sixty years, I was a nail biter. After just **one month** of taking red palm oil intermittently, the urge to bite my nails completely disappeared.

Now, three months later, I finally have stronger nails. For me, it was more than cosmetic—it was proof. Red palm oil calmed my nerves and restored brain balance.

"After sixty years of biting my nails, red palm oil gave me peace—and fingernails." My night vision is a little better and the floaters in my eyes are often gone too because I take selenium as well.

What quirks and habits do you notice in your family? The nervous tapping of a foot, the constant biting of nails, the mood swings that seem to run down the family tree, the child who struggles to focus, or the elder who battles brain fog.

Too often we cling to diagnoses, labels, and prescriptions as though they are the final words. We hold on to bad habits, old ways, and generational patterns without asking the deeper question: *what if these struggles are not permanent?*

What if healing, improvement, or even full restoration is possible—not by masking the symptoms, but by addressing the problem at its root?

Don't Cling to Labels or Diagnosis

Take a closer look at your family. Notice the quirks, the habits, the repeated struggles that seem to travel from one generation to the next. Is it the cousin who battles constant fatigue? The aunt who can't remember names? The nephew who can't sit still? The grandparents who drift into confusion? Or the special needs child with repetitive movements.

These are not random defects of character. They may be signs of missing nutrients, toxic exposures, or silent deficiencies passed down like unwanted heirlooms.

Do not cling to labels or diagnoses as if they are permanent. Too often I hear parents claim disease for themselves and a special need label for their children. You were never meant to be attached to a diagnosis. You are just supposed to hear the diagnosis, address and nourish it.

At its core, a diagnosis is simply your body's intelligent way of asking for what it needs. That request is for minerals that nourish and repair. Your brain is not broken— it is calling out for the tools to restore itself.

The request is simple yet powerful: step back, observe, and seek the root. **What you discover may not only heal you but also liberate generations to come.**

Simple Solutions

Bringing red palm oil into your family's life is simple:

- **For children:** 1 teaspoon twice a week can prevent Vitamin A deficiency.
- **For adults:** 1-2 tablespoons a week can provide antioxidants for eyes, heart, skin, and brain.
- **In the kitchen:** Stir into rice, drizzle into soups, after cooking.
- **For skin:** Apply as a natural lotion for deep moisture, sun protection, and healing support for eczema, rashes, or dryness.

You Have the Power

- Pregnant mothers and children under five are the most vulnerable to blindness from Vitamin A deficiency.
- But anyone, at any age, can lose their sight if deficiencies are ignored.
- Red palm oil, paired with selenium, protects both eyes and brain.

Dr. Llaila Afrika posits: "We see with our brain, not with our eyes." Feed the brain; sharpen the vision.

Mothers, grandmothers, sisters—you hold the power to stop blindness before it begins. Don't wait for institutions to tell you what you inherently know: *Food is medicine and Divine Intelligence is your guide.*

Vitamin E & Vision Protection

(The Guardian Nutrient)

What It Does

- Shields the **retina** and **lens** from oxidative stress that causes aging and clouding.
- Preserves the **lipid membranes** of eye cells and tiny retinal blood vessels.
- Works with **vitamins A and C** and **selenium** to neutralize damaging free radicals.

Where It Helps

- **Cataracts** slows oxidative lens damage.

- **Macular degeneration** helps protect retinal pigment cells.
- **Dry eyes / eye fatigue** supports healthy tear film and surface comfort.
- **Diabetic eye strain** aids micro-circulation and reduces inflammation.

Vitamin A & Vision Protection

- **Preventing night blindness-** (retinal function)
- **Maintaining corneal health and tear film**
- **Supporting mucous membranes** -of the eye
- **Reducing infection risk** -in ocular tissue
- **Dry eyes** -Restores epithelial health
- **Light sensitivity-** Improves retinal pigment health

Healing the Skin

The same nutrients that protect vision also **restore and renew the skin.** Applied topically, red palm oil becomes a soothing lotion and healing salve:

- **For babies:** gentle relief for diaper rash, cradle cap, and dry patches.
- **For children & teens:** calms eczema, nourishes sensitive skin, and supports healing of rashes and scars.
- **For adults:** locks in moisture, softens rough skin, and reduces the appearance of blemishes and stretch marks.

I added this section because I see so many mothers on social media inquiring how to heal their baby's skin and eczema.

From Skin to Hair: Beauty Beyond the Surface

What heals the skin often blesses the hair. The same **Vitamin A and Vitamin E** in red palm oil that soothe rashes and restore moisture also strengthen the scalp and crown.

A Crown of Health for Hair

Healthy hair is more than appearance—it is a reflection of inner and outer nourishment. Rich in **carotenoids, tocotrienols, and essential fats,** red palm oil fortifies hair from the root, restores shine to dull strands, and protects against damage.

Can we live without vitamin A?

No.

Sight, sound, and immunity depend on it. Life depends on it. Yet when red palm oil—nature's golden vessel of vitamin A—is named, fear rises where reverence should live. Be wary of voices that teach suspicion of the Earth's gifts. Nature was designed to nourish, not deceive.

CHAPTER 19 BIBLIOGRAPHY

Vitamin A — Eye & Vision

1. **World Health Organization.** *Vitamin A Deficiency: Xerophthalmia Spectrum (Night Blindness, Bitot's Spots, Corneal Xerosis, Ulceration, and Keratomalacia).* Geneva: World Health Organization, n.d.
2. **National Institutes of Health, Office of Dietary Supplements.** *Vitamin A: Health Professional Fact Sheet.* NIH, n.d.
3. **StatPearls Publishing.** "Xerophthalmia." *StatPearls*, 2024. https://www.statpearls.com.
4. **Community Eye Health Journal.** "The Eye Signs of Vitamin A Deficiency." *Community Eye Health Journal* 30, no. 98 (2017): 44–45.

Vitamin E — Retinal Protection & AMD Research

5. **National Eye Institute.** *AREDS and AREDS2 Clinical Trial Results.* National Institutes of Health, 2001–2013.
6. **Age-Related Eye Disease Study Research Group.** "A Randomized, Placebo-Controlled, Clinical Trial of High-Dose Supplementation with Vitamins C and E, Beta Carotene, and Zinc for Age-Related Macular Degeneration and Vision Loss." *Archives of Ophthalmology* 119, no. 10 (2001): 1417–1436.
7. **Various Authors.** "Reviews on Vitamin E in Age-Related Macular Degeneration and Retinal Protection: Tocopherols, Tocotrienols, and Oxidative Stress Pathways." *Ophthalmology Review Literature*, various years.
8. **Linus Pauling Institute, Oregon State University.** *Vitamin E (Tocopherols and Tocotrienols): Micronutrient Information Center.* Corvallis, OR: OSU, n.d.
9. **Recent Review.** "The Potential of Selenium-Based Therapies for Ocular Disease." *Ophthalmology & Vision Science Review* (2024).

10. **Antioxidants.** "Nutrients for Prevention of Macular Degeneration and Eye Diseases." *Antioxidants* 8, no. 9 (2019): Article 375.
11. **Ophthalmology Research Literature.** "Selenium-Dependent Antioxidant Defenses in Ocular Tissues." *JAMA Ophthalmology* and related journals, various years.
12. **Zeba, A. N., et al.** "Red Palm Oil Supplementation Improves Night Blindness in Children with Vitamin A Deficiency." *Nutrition Journal* 5 (2006): 20.

CHAPTER 20

SISTERS, ACTIVATE YOUR POWER: PREVENT HEARING LOSS

Vitamin A is one of the most powerful nutrients for protecting your hearing. For years, traditional diets rich in whole, unprocessed foods provided abundant vitamin A, while modern advice has often wrongly labeled it as "toxic." Yet research shows vitamin A is essential not only for vision, skin, and bone health, but also for **preventing and even reversing hearing loss.**

Historical and modern studies point to its importance:

- As early as **1823**, French researchers noticed that people who ate the most vitamin A-rich foods—along with vitamin B12 from sources like red meat—had better hearing.
- In **1984**, a European study reported that patients with age-related hearing loss improved their hearing by **5–15 decibels** when given vitamins A and E (found in foods like red palm oil).
- Other research shows that **vitamin A deficiency** reduces the number of sensory cells in the nose, tongue, and inner ear.
- A **1993 Science study** revealed that vitamin A can even stimulate the regeneration of auditory hair cells—the tiny structures responsible for hearing.
- In **2009**, Japanese scientists found that adults with the highest blood levels of vitamin A and carotenoids had the **lowest risk of hearing loss.**
- And in **2014**, researchers discovered that vitamin A deficiency during pregnancy—especially in the early stages—can predispose children to inner ear malformations and hearing problems later in life.

The evidence is clear: vitamin A not only supports good hearing, but may also help prevent tinnitus, regenerate damaged cells, and protect future generations.

CHAPTER 20 BIBLIOGRAPHY

Weston A. Price Foundation. "Vitamin A and Hearing Loss." Adapted from research reported by Bill Sardi, *Knowledge of Health*, May 21, 2014. Weston A. Price Foundation. https://www.westonaprice.org.

CHAPTER 21

NOSEBLEEDS – WHAT THE WEB WON'T CURE, MOTHER NATURE WILL

Each year, up to **60 million** people in the U.S. are estimated to have a nosebleed. *Your nose begins to bleed*. Or maybe your child runs up and says, *"Mommy, my nose is bleeding!"* Now what? Most of us go straight to the internet. The search results flood in…

"Pinch your nose, eat more leafy greens, don't pick your nose, use a humidifier, seek medical advice."

So, you try the advice you search on the internet. You pinch, you wait, you even run to the doctor. Yet for some of you, the nosebleeds continue—sometimes for years, sometimes for a lifetime.

Here's the trap: what was once a simple, natural imbalance has been captured, renamed, and medicalized. Your "nosebleed" was called *scurvy* in the past and *epistaxis* today.

Suddenly, the solution belongs to the medical industrial complex. These diagnoses feel unfamiliar, intimidating, and it sets you up to believe that only drugs, a doctor or surgery can solve your problem.

Instead of depending on Mother Nature, you become dependent on clinical definitions and prescriptions. These costs become your loss.

Why So Many Of Us Suffer

Nearly **200 million people** in this country will suffer from nosebleeds at some point, whether once or frequently according to research. I've met people who told me they had nosebleeds every single day!

Children are especially vulnerable. From ages 2 to 10, countless little ones experience nosebleeds. Adults over 50 may also face them more often. But the truth is: anyone, at any age, can have nosebleeds.

So, what can you do?

The Matriarchal Answer

The internet (artificial intelligence) won't tell you the full truth. Stop expecting AI to always give you the truth our mothers and grandmothers already knew: the answer to prevent nosebleeds was simply Vitamin C **gifts** from the earth:

Foods High in Vitamin C

(Nature's antioxidant shield — essential for immunity, iron absorption, collagen, skin, gums, and brain health)

Highest Vitamin C Sources (Superfoods)

These foods contain **more Vitamin C than oranges** and work beautifully for healing, immunity, and iron absorption:

Top 5 Vitamin C Foods (Real Power Sources)

1. **Habanero Pepper**
   ~100–220 mg Vitamin C per pepper
   One of the most concentrated, accessible vitamin C sources. Heat does **not** destroy its vitamin C.
2. **Guava**
   ~125–230 mg per cup
   High vitamin C + fiber. Excellent for immune and gut health.
3. **Kakadu Plum**
   ~2,000–3,000 mg per 100 g
   The **highest vitamin C food on Earth** (native to Australia).
4. **Blackcurrants**
   ~180 mg per cup
   Potent antioxidants plus immune-supporting flavonoids.
5. **Red Bell Pepper**
   ~190 mg per cup (raw)

Note: Vitamin C is not rare—it's concentrated in peppers, tropical fruits, and deeply pigmented plants. Even one habanero can deliver more vitamin C than several oranges combined.

*Vitamin C is **water-soluble**, meaning the body doesn't store it — you must refill it daily.*

Best Ways to Absorb Iron (with Vitamin C)

Vitamin C helps the body absorb iron more effectively—especially iron from plant foods.

To boost iron absorption:

- **Combine iron-rich foods with vitamin C–rich foods**
  (spinach + lemon, beans + tomatoes, lentils + peppers)
- **Avoid overcooking** vitamin C–rich foods, as vitamin C is sensitive to heat
- **Add vitamin C raw**: squeeze lemon or lime over vegetables, meats, or salads
- **Use natural powders** like Camu Camu or acerola for gentle daily support

Why Vitamin C Matters for Blood Vessels

Vitamin C plays a critical role in keeping blood vessels **strong and flexible**. It helps the body make **collagen**, which reinforces the walls of veins and capillaries.

When vitamin C is **chronically low**:

- Blood vessels can become fragile
- Bruising may occur more easily
- Nosebleeds or gum bleeding may become more common
- Healing slows

Foods rich in vitamin C act as a **natural shield**, helping protect blood vessels and support healthy circulation.

Two weeks ago, my 10-year-old granddaughter had a nosebleed. This wasn't her first. Instead of panicking, I reached for what Mother Nature already provided. I gave her a Vitamin C tablet and said, *"By the time you get upstairs, the bleeding will stop."* And it did. Quickly. Naturally and without fear. This just means she hasn't had any vitamin C rich foods for several days.

When Vitamin C is low, the entire body begins to struggle:

- **Bleeding begins inside and out.** Your nose, gums, and even internal organs can bleed—but you have the power to stop the bleeding by restoring Vitamin C.
- **Collagen breaks down.** Without Vitamin C, the body can't build or repair collagen, the protein that holds your skin, blood vessels, bones, and organs together.
- **Blood vessels weaken.** Capillaries become fragile, causing easy bruising and unexplained bleeding.
- **Gums swell and bleed.** Teeth may loosen because the tissue holding them in place begins to break down.
- **Wounds heal slowly.** Cuts, sores, and skin injuries struggle to close. Fatigue, weakness, and joint pain begin to appear.
- **Anemia develops.** Bleeding plus poor iron absorption leads to low iron levels—and deep exhaustion.

Vitamin C is not optional. It is daily, foundational nutrition—your body's natural medicine for *healing,* ***sealing,*** *strengthening, and repairing.*

On A Personal Note

I keep Camu Camu Vitamin C in a jar but I mix it with MSM. Most days, I take a teaspoon in water at least once a day.

MSM is widely used to support connective tissue and help the body process environmental burdens, including residues from pesticides. Dr. Afrika often reminded us that pesticide and roach spray are essentially the same thing—call it what you want, but its purpose is to kill bugs.

The problem is not just exposure; it's **accumulation**. Over time, these chemicals lodge in tissues, contributing to pain, stiffness, blockages, and chronic irritation.

MSM is commonly paired with **vitamin C**, which supports collagen formation and antioxidant defense. Together, they are often used to help reduce inflammation and discomfort associated with environmental stressors.

I've seen this combination make a difference firsthand.

My spiritual sister, Padiyah E Pelle, kept complaining to me about leg pain—no injury, no clear cause. I told her to try vitamin C with MSM. Three days later, she called and said, *"Guess what? My leg pain is gone."*

I had my own moment of clarity with this pair. Persistent rotator cuff pain had been limiting my movement. I began taking MSM with **organic camu camu vitamin**

C, mixed together in a large glass jar. I took one teaspoon daily. In less than 3 days, the pain eased and mobility returned.

My son reaches for tangerines—bright, living vitamin C in his hands. There are many doors to the same house: fruit, powders, teas, tonics. Choose the habit you'll keep. I honor both—fruit for the life it carries, supplements for the steadiness they bring—so the body remembers, the mind stays clear, and the day begins already nourished.

These are not miracles—they are reminders.

The most powerful routines are often the simplest ones: practices you can do **every single day**, straight from your kitchen. When something is visible, easy to prepare, and easy to remember, it becomes sustainable. And sustainability is where healing habits live.

Time to Return to Wisdom

Be mindful when you conduct research—especially with artificial intelligence. The answers you receive are often fragments, not the full truth. These tools can point you in a direction, but they rarely reveal the whole picture. Always dig deeper, cross-check, and use your own wisdom as the final filter.

We cannot live without vitamin C. Without it, blood vessels weaken, tissues break down, and bleeding follows. Yet most medical labs don't check it. Nosebleeds, bleeding gums, and easy bruising are not normal—they are warning signs. Vitamin C is essential. Take it.

CHAPTER 21 BIBLIOGRAPHY

1. **Hemilä, H.** "Vitamin C and the Common Cold." *British Journal of Nutrition* 67, no. 1 (1992): 3–16.
   Carr, A., and S. Maggini. "Vitamin C and Immune Function." *Nutrients* 9, no. 11 (2017): 1211.
2. **Paterson, C. R.** "Vitamin C and Capillary Fragility." *The Lancet* 314, no. 8146 (1979): 1426–1427.
3. **National Institutes of Health, Office of Dietary Supplements.** *Vitamin C Fact Sheet for Consumers*. NIH, n.d.
4. **Yale Medicine.** "Nosebleeds (Epistaxis)." *Yale Medicine*, n.d. https://www.yalemedicine.org/conditions/epistaxis.

CHAPTER 22

VITAMIN E IS NOT A LUXURY — IT'S A HEALER!

The Nutrient You Can't Live Without

Imagine your body as a living city where tiny sparks sometimes fly. Most of these sparks come from molecules like hydrogen peroxide — a natural signal your body uses to communicate, call for help, and trigger healing.

In small amounts, hydrogen peroxide is a messenger. But when too many sparks fly at once, they stop sending signals and start burning things down. That's when free radicals begin jumping from cell to cell, stealing electrons and creating damage.

Vitamin E for Migraines and Seizures

Vitamin E slows the aging process, protects the nerves, and brings relief from migraines and headaches. It strengthens every arm of the immune system, helping your body block infections before they take hold.

When vitamin E is low, skin becomes fragile and slow to repair. Wounds linger. Scars deepen. Rashes, eczema, and shingles grow more severe. Uterine recovery slows, and even seizures can flare in a body starving for this essential nutrient.

Vitamin E restores what life has worn down—and it protects what future generations will depend on.

Because vitamin E is the skin's frontline antioxidant, chronically low levels mean more UV damage and a higher risk of certain skin cancers. Yet its hidden power runs even deeper. Vitamin E supports male potency, protects the prostate from inflammation, strengthens female fertility, eases cramps and menstrual disorders, improves outcomes after miscarriage, and supports healthy lactation.

When Deficiency Turns Deadly

Hydrogen peroxide is one of the body's earliest distress signals. It tells white blood cells exactly where to go in the body to repair damaged tissues, fight infections, and clean up injuries. After the work is done, **Vitamin E steps in to calm the storm**—helping hydrogen peroxide break down into harmless water and oxygen so it can leave the body.

But what happens when your Vitamin E stores are empty?

Hydrogen peroxide builds up in the wrong places. Oxidative stress rises. Tissues become irritated, inflamed, and slow to heal.

Symptoms we label as "disease" often begin as nothing more than a **silent, long-term Vitamin E deficiency**—a missing antioxidant that should have been there to restore balance.

- Fluid buildup around the lungs → **Asthma**
- Fluid buildup around the heart → **Congestive heart failure**
- Fluid buildup in the gut → **Colitis that becomes chronic**
- Fluid in the brain → **Seizures**

If hydrogen peroxide builds up too long, it transforms into **free radicals**—tiny "wrecking balls" that smash into your cells, tearing them apart. First, your body begs for Vitamin E's help. But when none comes, the fluid and destruction spreads. And in my opinion, I believe this has a lot to do with strokes and sepsis.

Vitamin E doesn't just support healing—without it, the body cannot complete the healing cycle at all.

This is why people with **HIV, cancer, liver disease, kidney problems, or heart disease** often get worse faster. The real killer is unchecked oxidative stress—the very thing Vitamin E was designed to protect us from.

Infants, children, and adults are suffering because essentials go missing. Here, we are witnessing what happens when **vitamin E—one of nature's great guardians—is not stored and renewed.**

Red palm oil contains the **full Vitamin E spectrum** (tocopherols and tocotrienols), plus extra antioxidants like carotenoids that make its power even stronger. For thousands of years, cultures across Africa and beyond have used red palm oil for food, medicine, and healing. Pregnant women and new mothers took it to protect their health and their babies.

The real tragedy isn't that disease exists - we chase complicated answers, while the solution is right in front of us.

Why Most Vitamin E Supplements Are Incomplete

Vitamin E is not one vitamin — it is a **family of eight nutrients**:
4 Tocopherols

- **α-tocopherol (alpha)
- β-tocopherol (beta)
- γ-tocopherol (gamma)
- δ-tocopherol (delta)**

4 Tocotrienols

- **α-tocotrienol
- β-tocotrienol
- γ-tocotrienol
- δ-tocotrienol**

Together, they form the **full spectrum** of Vitamin E that the body uses for:

- antioxidant protection
- brain and nerve protection
- fertility
- immune function
- heart and liver health
- thyroid and selenium synergy

But here's the problem:
Most store-bought Vitamin E supplements contain only alpha-tocopherol.
That's **1 out of 8** forms.

Why This Is a Problem

Research shows that taking **only alpha-tocopherol**:

- **reduces your body's gamma-tocopherol levels** (a major protector against inflammation and toxins)
- **blocks tocotrienols**, which are *far* more powerful antioxidants
- **creates imbalance**, not full nourishment

This is like giving the body **one violinist and calling it an orchestra.**
**Tocopherol-only Vitamin E = half an engine.
Tocotrienols + tocopherols = the full engine.

The Better Choice: Full-Spectrum Vitamin E

The richest natural sources of full-spectrum Vitamin E are:

- **Red palm oil (highest in tocotrienols)**
- **Wheat germ oil**
- Annatto (gamma- and delta-tocotrienols)
- Sunflower seeds
- Almonds
- Hazelnuts
- Avocado

What Tocotrienols Can Do

- **Protect the brain:** They keep brain cells safe from damage and may reduce the risk of memory loss, dementia, and Alzheimer's.
- **Fight cancer:** They stop dangerous cancer cells from growing too fast and help the body get rid of them.
- **Build strong bones:** They help keep bones from becoming weak and brittle.
- **Balance blood sugar:** For people with diabetes, they can help keep blood sugar under control.
- **Protect the liver and stomach:** They defend against fatty liver disease and keep the gut healthy.
- **Support the heart:** They improve cholesterol and keep blood vessels flexible.

The Oldest Naturally Occurring Vitamin E and A In One Palm Tree

Red palm oil just may be the **oldest source of full-spectrum Vitamin E** on the planet.

- It contains both tocopherols and all tocotrienols.
- It includes extra antioxidants like carotene that boost its healing power.
- It has been trusted in traditional diets for thousands of years.

Red Palm Oil vs. Oxidized Palm Oil

About half of palm oil is made up of **saturated fats**, but interestingly, it does not cause the same heart problems (like clogged arteries or blood clots) that other saturated fats can.

Palm oil has a good balance of **saturated and unsaturated fats**, and it is rich in natural antioxidants like **beta-carotene** (the same nutrient that makes carrots orange) and **vitamin E**. These nutrients help protect the body from damage.

Studies show that while palm oil can raise cholesterol a little more than some other oils (like corn or soybean oil), it also helps the body lower its own cholesterol production. This may be because of special nutrients in palm oil called **tocotrienols** and the way its fatty acids are arranged.

Health benefits of palm oil include:

- Lower risk of blood clots and clogged arteries.
- Helping control blood pressure.
- Supporting healthy red blood cells and immune function.

The problem: When palm oil is **fresh** or made into red palm oil, it can be good for you. But when it becomes oxidized (damaged by heat and processing), it can be harmful. Oxidized palm oil has been linked to problems with the heart, liver, lungs, kidneys, and even reproduction.

So, eating moderate amounts of fresh or red palm oil may support good health, but eating too much, or eating oxidized palm oil can be dangerous. Because it contains beta-carotene, red palm oil may also help protect against vitamin A deficiency and possibly some forms of cancer.

In simple words: Fresh palm oil can be healthy in small amounts, but *old or overheated* palm oil can hurt the body. This is why we add palm oil to a biscuit, or in a bowl of cooked rice, cooked soups or cooked oatmeal.

Personally, I avoid cooking with palm oil. Instead, I add it to my bowl of soup. My son adds palm oil to his bowl of oatmeal twice a week.

Palm Oil: The Good vs. Oxidized

- Rich in antioxidants (beta-carotene, vitamin E)
- Helps lower body's own cholesterol production
- May reduce risk of clogged arteries and blood clots
- Supports healthy blood pressure
- Improves immune function and red blood cells
- May protect against vitamin A deficiency and some **cancers**

Oxidized Palm Oil (damaged by heat and processing)

- Raises "bad" cholesterol (unhealthy lipid profile)
- Can harm the heart, liver, lungs, and kidneys
- May cause reproductive problems
- Leads to toxic byproducts in the body
- Linked to cell damage in the liver

What Does "Processed" Mean for Palm Oil?

Palm oil doesn't come out of the fruit ready for the bottle. It usually goes through **processing** — steps that change its color, flavor, texture, or shelf life. Some processing is gentle and keeps nutrients, but heavy processing (like too much heat or chemical treatment) can make the oil **oxidized** and less healthy.

Signs Palm Oil is Processed / Oxidized

- Fresh red palm oil is naturally **red-orange** because of beta-carotene. If the oil looks clear or yellowish like vegetable oil, it has usually been processed heavily.
- **Very long shelf life** → If it can sit on a shelf for years without spoiling, it has likely been refined a lot. *Remember palm comes from the fruit of the palm tree.*
- **Labeled as "refined," "bleached," or "deodorized"** → These words mean it has gone through chemical or high-heat processing.
- **Used in packaged foods** → If you see "palm oil" or "vegetable oil" in cookies, chips, instant noodles, or fast food, it's almost always **heavily processed** palm oil.

Signs Palm Oil is Fresh / Healthier

- **Red palm oil** → Keeps its natural reddish-orange color from beta-carotene.
- **Cold-pressed or minimally processed** → Labels that say "virgin," "unrefined," or "cold-pressed" mean less heat and more nutrients are kept.
- **Sold in health food stores** → Usually marketed as "red palm oil" with info about vitamin E and carotenoid.
-

Simple rule:

- Red, unrefined (may appear orange) = better for health.
- Clear color refined = more processed, less healthy.

Note: Can we live without Vitamin E? **No!** We cannot live without vitamin E because it protects our cells, brain, nerves, and immune system from oxidative damage. Without vitamin E, tissues break down faster than the body can repair them, leading to inflammation, nerve damage, and weakened immunity. Vitamin E works with vitamins A and C, selenium, and healthy fats to preserve life and longevity.

CHAPTER 22 BIBLIOGRAPHY

1. **Traber, M. G., and J. Atkinson.** "Vitamin E: Antioxidant and Nothing More." *Free Radical Biology and Medicine* 43, no. 1 (2007): 4–15. https://doi.org/10.1016/j.freeradbiomed.2007.03.024.
2. **Traber, M. G.** "Vitamin E Inadequacy in Humans: Causes and Consequences." *Advances in Nutrition* 5, no. 5 (2014): 503–514. https://doi.org/10.3945/an.114.006254.
3. **Jiang, Q.** "Natural Forms of Vitamin E: Metabolism, Antioxidant, and Anti-Inflammatory Activities and Their Role in Disease Prevention and Therapy." *Free Radical Biology and Medicine* 72 (2014): 76–90. https://doi.org/10.1016/j.freeradbiomed.2014.03.035.
4. **Aggarwal, B. B., C. Sundaram, S. Prasad, and R. Kannappan.** "Tocotrienols, the Vitamin E of the 21st Century: Its Potential Against Cancer and Other Chronic Diseases." *Biochemical Pharmacology* 80, no. 11 (2010): 1613–1631. https://doi.org/10.1016/j.bcp.2010.07.043.

5. **Sen, C. K., S. Khanna, and S. Roy.** "Tocotrienols: Vitamin E Beyond Tocopherols." *Life Sciences* 78, no. 18 (2007): 2088–2098. https://doi.org/10.1016/j.lfs.2005.12.001.
6. **Peh, H. Y., W. S. D. Tan, W. Liao, and W. S. F. Wong.** "Vitamin E Therapy Beyond Cancer: Tocopherol versus Tocotrienol." *Pharmacology & Therapeutics* 162 (2016): 152–169. https://doi.org/10.1016/j.pharmthera.2015.12.003.
7. **Fu, J. Y., H. L. Che, D. M. Tan, and K. T. Teng.** "Bioavailability of Tocotrienols: Evidence in Human Studies." *Nutrition & Metabolism* 11, no. 1 (2014): 5. https://doi.org/10.1186/1743-7075-11-5.
8. **Rimm, E. B., M. J. Stampfer, A. Ascherio, E. Giovannucci, G. A. Colditz, and W. C. Willett.** "Vitamin E Consumption and the Risk of Coronary Heart Disease in Men." *New England Journal of Medicine* 328, no. 20 (1993): 1450–1456. https://doi.org/10.1056/NEJM199305203282004.
9. **Zainal, Z., et al.** "Therapeutic Potential of Palm Oil Vitamin E–Derived Tocotrienols: Anti-Inflammation, Antioxidant Activity, Nutritional Supplementation, and Clinical Evidence." *Food Research International* (2022). https://doi.org/10.1016/j.foodres.2022.111175.
10. **Gopalan, Y., I. L. Shuaib, E. Magosso, et al.** "Clinical Investigation of the Protective Effects of Palm Tocotrienols on Brain White Matter." *Stroke* 45, no. 5 (2014): 1422–1428. https://doi.org/10.1161/STROKEAHA.113.004449.
11. **Sen, C. K., S. Khanna, C. Rink, and S. Roy.** "Tocotrienols: The Emerging Face of Natural Vitamin E." *Molecular Aspects of Medicine* 28, nos. 5–6 (2007): 692–728. https://doi.org/10.1016/j.mam.2007.07.001

CHAPTER 23

THERE IS NO 'US' WITHOUT SELENIUM

In many parts of the United States—the Northeast, Southeast, Northwest, and Southwest—the soil is low in selenium. When the soil is empty, the food is empty. Fruits, vegetables, and grains grown there carry only a fraction of what the heart, brain, and immune system truly need.

Selenium is a tiny mineral with giant responsibilities. It guards life, immunity, and protection. People and animals cannot thrive without it. Our cancers, heart problems, and cognitive decline are telling us the truth: we are not receiving our rightful share of selenium.

Why Selenium Matters

Selenium:

- Helps lower the risk of certain cancers, heart problems, thyroid issues, and brain diseases.
- Prevents problems caused by low levels—fatigue, weakness, and difficulty thinking clearly.
- Is the backbone of selenoproteins, the enzymes that shield cells from damage and oxidation.

When selenium is missing, every system suffers: immunity weakens, the heart strains, the brain slows, and the thyroid can no longer keep up.

What Dr. Gerhard Schrauzer Discovered

The late Dr. Gerhard N. Schrauzer—was a chemist, professor at UC San Diego, Nobel Prize nominator, and pioneer of selenium research—spent his life tracing one pattern:

Low selenium, high disease.
Adequate selenium, lower disease.

Across 27 countries, he found an inverse relationship between selenium intake and cancer deaths:

- Populations with **300–350 mcg/day** of selenium had far lower rates of breast, lung, prostate, and colon cancer.
- Populations living on **50–100 mcg/day** saw cancer rise without mercy.
- Australians averaged **~100 mcg/day**.
- Japanese nearly **300 mcg/day**.
- Meanwhile, the U.S. recommendation stayed at **55–70 mcg/day**—a level Schrauzer knew was dangerously low for real cancer protection.

Breast Cancer Study

In one kibbutz study, the research team found serum selenium dropping as breast cancer advanced:

- Stage 1: ~10 mcg
- Stage 2: ~9 mcg
- Stage 3: ~8 mcg
- Stage 4: ~8 mcg

As selenium reserves fell, cancer severity deepened—proof that deficiency is not a side note, but a driver.

Stories that Should Have Changed Medicine

Lymphedema

At a conference, Dr. Schrauzer noticed a woman with severe lymphedema—her arm swollen, blistered, and inflamed months after breast surgery. He gave her **800 mcg of sodium selenite**.

Within about 40 minutes, the redness faded and the swelling softened. By morning, her arm was nearly normal.

He went on to study 86 other women with lymphedema and saw the same pattern: selenium reduced swelling and inflammation. Europe now recognizes selenium as a support therapy for lymphedema.

Note: In emergencies Schrauzer relied on sodium selenite. For everyday use he favored nutritional yeast-based selenium.

Athlete's Heart / Keshan Disease

As a young man, Schrauzer struggled with running. A college exam revealed an enlarged heart—what they called an "athlete's heart." It was actually the early stage of **Keshan disease**, a selenium-deficiency cardiomyopathy.

Schrauzer grew up in a spa region famous for healing waters—but the soil around his town was selenium-poor. Once Schrauzer received adequate selenium, his swollen 'athlete's' heart returned to normal size. Deficiency had enlarged it; selenium helped restore it.

Septicemia, Pneumonia, Stroke, Pancreatitis

European studies showed that selenium:

- Reduced deaths from **septicemia**, especially when **pneumonia** was present.
- Lessened **stroke-related brain damage**, by protecting neurons.
- Lowered mortality in **acute pancreatitis**, a condition often considered hopeless.

From the *ICU to the recovery ward*, one truth kept emerging: when selenium was restored, outcomes improved.

Vision

The eyes naturally store high levels of selenium. Animal research confirms species with sharp vision often have more selenium in their eyes – like cats for example, they have high concentrations of selenium in their eyes which is why they can see well.

In human studies, about **80%** of patients reported vision improvement after selenium supplementation. Schrauzer himself went from worrying about his California driver's test in his 30s to no longer needing glasses after he began taking selenium regularly.

Selenium Across the Lifespan

Thyroid

The thyroid makes T4, but it is selenium-dependent enzymes that convert T4 into active **T3**. Without selenium, thyroid hormones stay "half-asleep," and the body drifts into fatigue, weight gain, and slowed thinking.

AIDS/HIV and Immunity

Schrauzer was among the first to recommend selenium for people living with HIV/AIDS. Studies showed:

- Improved symptoms with selenium supplementation.
- Lower rates of cardiomyopathy (heart muscle damage).
- Reduced depression when selenium was restored.

He saw again and again without selenium, the immune system cannot do its job.

Liver Damage & Alcohol

In animal studies, selenium-deficient diets caused lethal liver necrosis in just two weeks. In people, a severely alcoholic man with almost no selenium in his blood made a remarkable recovery after high-dose selenium support.

Infants & Children

In Western nations and Australia, infants often experience a steep drop in selenium status during the first 4–5 months of life. Levels can approach deficiency before slowly climbing back.

Japanese infants **do not** experience this steep decline—they maintain higher selenium reserves from birth. Schrauzer concluded: On the other hand, Western selenium intake is too low to protect babies fully.

When infants lack selenium:

- Their **immune system** weakens.
- The **heart** is more vulnerable.
- The **thyroid** slows energy and growth.
- The **brain** misses critical protection during development.

Schrauzer believed children should receive **20–50 mcg/day**, and teenagers even more, based on their size and growth.

Pregnancy & Placental Health

Veterinary medicine long ago proved it: without *selenium*, animals suffer miscarriages and **retained placenta**—a costly and dangerous complication.

Selenium helps prevent this in livestock, and Schrauzer believed the same logic applies to human mothers. He recommended **200–300 mcg/day** in pregnancy to protect both mother and child and to keep the placenta moving as it should after birth.

What Selenium Deficiency Looks Like

Selenium deficiency is not rare—it is **silent**. Common signs include:

- Frequent colds, infections, or slow recovery
- Fatigue, weight gain, or hair loss
- Brain fog, memory problems, mood swings
- Muscle weakness or cramps
- Fertility struggles or pregnancy complications
- **Enlarged heart** or cardiomyopathy

At the extreme, deficiency can lead to Keshan disease—a dilated cardiomyopathy born directly from low selenium in the soil and food. The heart enlarges, weakens, and may fail, while the label "heart disease" is written on the chart and the word "selenium" is never spoken.

I tell my readers:

- If your heart beats **slow**, consider iodine.
- If your heart beats **irregularly**, consider selenium.

In parts of China, even one-year-olds receive selenium to protect their hearts. They see deficiency as a cause. In America, we often never hear the word selenium.

How Much Is Enough?

Schrauzer's selenium research indicates:

- **55 mcg/day** (the U.S. RDA) is **too low** for real cancer protection.
- **75 mcg/day** may still be inadequate to replenish what the body uses.
- **200–300 mcg/day** for adults offers stronger protection, especially against cancer.
- The **upper safe limit** is generally recognized as **400 mcg/day**, especially when sourced from nutritional forms.

Schrauzer personally took **300–400 mcg/day** for over 30 years.

Important: Individual needs vary. Illness, medications, and other conditions matter. Always discuss dose decisions with a qualified health professional.

Sick people often need more selenium because their bodies burn through it faster. Fighting infection, inflammation, and oxidative damage consumes selenium-dependent enzymes at a high rate.

Forms of Selenium: When and Why

1. Sodium Selenite (Inorganic)

- A synthetic salt used in hospital IV nutrition and some fortification programs.
- Absorbed quickly, useful for **short-term, acute** situations (like lymphedema or parenteral feeding).
- Higher toxicity risk if misused; not ideal for daily, long-term supplementation.

2. Selenium Yeast / Selenomethionine (Organic)

- Yeast grown in selenium-rich medium; the yeast turns inorganic selenium into **organic selenomethionine**.
- Highly bioavailable and stored in tissues like an amino acid.
- Safer and gentler for **everyday use**, thyroid health, and long-term protection.

In simple terms:

- **Sodium selenite** – for clinical/emergency settings, under supervision.
- **Selenium yeast** – for daily wellness and prevention.

Food Sources & Their Limits

- **SelenoExcell selenium yeast** – my personal, consistent preference.
- **Oyster-based supplements** – can supply selenium, iodine, copper, and zinc in one.
- **Brazil nuts** – powerful but unpredictable. Selenium content varies widely by soil and country of origin. One nut may deliver a lot; another very little.

Other foods like garlic, onions, mushrooms, broccoli, tomatoes, radishes, Swiss chard, and astragalus can also contain selenium—**only if** the soil does. In large parts of America, it doesn't.

So, if you eat local food grown on low-selenium soil, your diet will reflect that emptiness. That is why supplementation often becomes essential.

Selenium works even better with **full-spectrum Vitamin E**—from sources like wheat germ oil or red palm oil—to build a strong antioxidant shield.

Selenium, Place, and Survival

Where you live matters.

- In Keshan County, China, ultra-low soil selenium led to Keshan disease—heart failure driven by deficiency. Once people received selenium, the disease nearly disappeared.
- In some regions of Italy and China, doctors were trained to **prescribe selenium** where soil was poor. Italy went further, with iodine programs and a ban on potassium bromate.

In the U.S., we rarely hear that kind of proactive prevention. Our people pay the price with pacemakers, heart transplants, and cognitive decline—solutions that treat damage, not deficiency.

The documentary stories of **Blue Zones** echoes the same wisdom. An Italian man left the U.S., moved near the sea, planted his vineyard, and lived decades beyond his "*six-month" cancer prognosis*? His life was quietly held up another 30 plus years by sunlight, soil minerals, sea proximity, and a simpler, nutrient-dense diet—things our current system rarely honors.

Front Line Warriors

You may never have heard the name **Gerhard Schrauzer**, but his work has likely already touched your life or hopefully it will soon.

He stood shoulder to shoulder with lawyers like **Jonathan Emord** and advocates chronicled in **WholeFoods Magazine**, fighting for the right to share truthful scientific claims about nutrients and disease—against strong resistance by the FDA.

Because of these warriors, we are still allowed to read and speak about selenium's role in cancer, heart disease, immunity, and brain health.

The Takeaway: Begin with What's Missing

Selenium is not a wellness "extra." It is a cornerstone of:

- Longevity
- Vitality
- Resilience

When you are searching for the roots of your family's health struggles, ask first: **What is missing?**

- Is the soil empty?
- Is the plate empty?
- Is the heart starved of selenium?
- Is the thyroid asking for both iodine and selenium?

Begin by restoring what the earth was meant to give you: selenium, iodine, and their supporting nutrients. Replace deficiency with sufficiency. Let the selenoproteins turn back on.

Note: Because there truly is **no "us" without selenium**—no strong hearts, no sharp minds, no resilient immunity, no steady future. This page was meant to give you the tools to fight for your health.

CHAPTER 23 BIBLIOGRAPHY

1. **Schrauzer, G. N.** (1988). *Selenium: Present Status and Perspectives in Biology and Medicine.* Humana Press. **Schrauzer, Gerhard N.**, ed. *Selenium.* Berlin: Springer-Verlag, 1978.
2. **Schrauzer, Gerhard N.** "Selenium and Cancer: A Review." *Bioinorganic Chemistry* 7, no. 1 (1977): 23–34.
3. **Schrauzer, Gerhard N., and Daniel T. Lee.** "Selenium and Breast Cancer: Clinical and Laboratory Evidence." *Biological Trace Element Research* 49, no. 1 (1995): 1–7.
4. **Schrauzer, Gerhard N.** "Selenomethionine: A Review of Its Nutritional Significance." *Journal of Nutrition* 133, no. 5 (2003): 1453S–1456S.
5. **Schrauzer, Gerhard N.** "Selenium in the Prevention of Human Cancers." *Journal of the American College of Nutrition* 17, no. 1 (1998): 12–27.
6. **American Journal of Clinical Nutrition.** "Selenium Status and Cardiomyopathy: Keshan Disease." *AJCN* Special Report, 1994.
7. **Yang, Gonghuan, et al.** "The Relationship Between Selenium and Keshan Disease." *Biomedical and Environmental Sciences* 1, no. 3 (1988): 199–210.
8. **McKenzie, Robert C., and Michael P. Rayman.** "Thyroid Hormone Metabolism and Selenium." *Thyroid* 9, no. 8 (1999): 761–767.
9. **Rayman, Margaret P.** "Selenium and Human Health." *The Lancet* 379, no. 9822 (2012): 1256–1268.
10. **Flohé, L., and W. A. Günzler.** "Glutathione Peroxidase." *Methods in Enzymology* 105 (1984): 114–121.
11. **Dworkin, B., et al.** "Selenium Deficiency in Alcoholic Cirrhosis." *Hepatology* 9, no. 3 (1989): 473–478.
12. **Kupka, R., et al.** "Selenium Status, Immune Function, and HIV." *Journal of Nutrition* 134, no. 10 (2004): 3022–3026.
13. **Baum, M. K., et al.** "Selenium and HIV Disease Progression." *Journal of Acquired Immune Deficiency Syndromes* 33, no. 5 (2003): 501–508.
14. **Kiremidjian-Schumacher, L., and R. M. Roy.** "Selenium and Immune Function." *International Reviews of Immunology* 17, no. 2–3 (1998): 123–148.
15. **Clark, L. C., et al.** "Effects of Selenium Supplementation for Cancer Prevention in Patients with Carcinoma of the Skin." *JAMA* 276, no. 24 (1996): 1957–1963.
16. **Mayo Clinic Proceedings.** "Lymphedema Treatment and Selenium Therapy." *MCP*, 1995–2003.

17. **Kasseroller, R. G.** "Selenium in the Treatment of Secondary Lymphedema." *Pflege Zeitschrift* 48, no. 6 (1995): 391–394.
18. **USDA Agricultural Research Service.** *US Soil Selenium Distribution Map.* Washington, DC: U.S. Department of Agriculture, 2001.
19. **National Research Council.** *Selenium in Nutrition.* Washington, DC: National Academy Press, 1983.
20. **Wen, Hong, et al.** "Selenium Status in Infants: Geographic Variation and Early Declines." *European Journal of Clinical Nutrition* 56, no. 11 (2002): 993–998.
21. **Robinson, M. F.** "Selenium in Human Pregnancy." *American Journal of Clinical Nutrition* 46, no. 2 (1987): 230–236.
22. **Schwarz, K., and C. M. Foltz.** "Selenium as an Integral Part of Factor 3 Against Dietary Necrotic Liver Degeneration." *Journal of Nutrition* 62, no. 2 (1957): 231–245.
23. **Finley, J. W.** "Bioavailability of Selenium from Foods." *Nutrition Reviews* 63, no. 3 (2005): 73–79.
24. **Hurst, R., et al.** "Selenium Intake and Brazil Nuts: Variability and Risks." *Journal of Nutrition* 140, no. 4 (2010): 795–800.
25. **Burk, Raymond F., and Gladys N. Hill.** "Selenoprotein P: A Selenium-Rich Plasma Protein." *Journal of Nutrition* 125, no. 7 (1995): 1438–1443.
26. **World Health Organization.** *Selenium in Human Health and Development.* Geneva: WHO Micronutrient Series, 2004.
27. **Rayman, Margaret P.** "Food-Chain Selenium and Human Disease." *Annual Review of Nutrition* 22 (2002): 215–245.
28. **Dos Reis, Manoela A., et al.** "Soil Selenium Deficiency and Human Health: A Review." *Environmental Geochemistry and Health* 39, no. 4 (2017): 1049–1073.
29. **Schrauzer, Gerhard N.** "*Interview by Natural Health Journalist Blake Graham.*" YouTube, December 23, 2022. Video, 54:29. https://youtu.be/Av4sg0zMe6o.

CHAPTER 24

A POWER PAIR: IODINE AND SELENIUM

Some nutrients are powerful on their own. Others reveal their true strength only when they work together. **Iodine and selenium are one such pair**—designed to function in harmony to regulate thyroid health, metabolism, energy, immune defense, and brain function.

Separating them weakens their full potential.

Iodine is essential for the production of thyroid hormones—the master regulators of growth, metabolism, reproduction, and energy.

Selenium is the guardian that activates and balances those hormones. Without selenium, iodine cannot be properly used. Without iodine, selenium has no hormones to protect.

If you or a family member experience symptoms such as memory loss, major mood changes, slow thinking, fatigue, a swollen neck, new tremors, or fertility challenges, consult a licensed clinician and ask about **thyroid testing**, **urinary iodine**, and/or **serum selenium levels**.

We now understand what happens to children when their brains are deprived of iodine and selenium. But what happens—quietly and over time—when **adult brains** go without them?

When left unprotected, the adult brain slows. People develop hypothyroid-like changes: sluggish thinking, memory lapses, depression, and fatigue. The ability to learn, plan, and adapt gradually erodes. Over time, the risk of neurodegenerative decline and poor recovery from injury increases.

Selenium, iodine, and vitamin E can support brain health and may help reduce risk, slow progression, or improve resilience in neurodegenerative disease—but **they are not cures**.

Neurodegenerative diseases include:

- **Alzheimer's disease** – affects memory, thinking, and behavior
- **Parkinson's disease** – affects movement, balance, and coordination
- **ALS (Amyotrophic Lateral Sclerosis)** – weakens muscles and breathing
- **Huntington's disease** – causes movement, mood, and cognitive decline
- **Multiple sclerosis (MS)** – damages nerve coverings, affecting strength and vision
- **Frontotemporal dementia** – affects personality, behavior, and language
- **Vascular dementia** – caused by reduced blood flow to the brain

Iodine and selenium are complementary teammates. When one is missing, the other cannot do its job.
One builds. The other protects.
Together, iodine and selenium allow the thyroid to work powerfully—and safely. Together, they help the heart beat steadily and the brain process information with clarity and speed.

Signs of Combined Iodine and Selenium Deficiency

When both are lacking, the body signals distress:

- **Puffiness or swelling** (especially under the eyes or ankles) — selenium supports albumin, which helps regulate fluid balance
- **Goiter or neck fullness** — iodine deficiency causes the thyroid to enlarge
- **Persistent fatigue and coldness** — slowed metabolism and heartbeat
- **Weight gain and sluggish metabolism**
- **Brain fog and slow thinking**
- **Impairs metabolic signaling,** contributing to sluggish glucose handling and energy imbalance.

The Trio: Iodine, Selenium, and Vitamin E

Iodine should not be taken alone—it needs selenium. Selenium, in turn, works best alongside **vitamin E**, especially in full-spectrum forms.
This trio:

- Energizes the thyroid
- Neutralizes free radicals
- Strengthens immune and brain defenses

Wheat Germ Oil (Tocopherols)

- Rich in α-tocopherol
- Supports fertility, skin repair, and hormonal balance
- Stable and nourishing

Red Palm Oil (Tocotrienols)

- Rich in α- and γ-tocotrienols
- Penetrates tissues rapidly
- Exceptional for brain, heart, and cellular repair

In short:

- **Wheat germ oil = classic vitamin E**
- **Red palm oil = advanced vitamin E**

Together, they complete the same kind of partnership as **iodine and selenium**.

Key Benefits Side-by-Side

Benefit Category	*Wheat Germ Oil*	*Red Palm Oil*
Vitamin E Type	High in α-tocopherol	Very high in tocotrienols
Brain Protection	Moderate	**Excellent — neuroprotective, improves nerve signaling**
Heart Health	Stabilizes cholesterol	**Reduces arterial plaque, lowers inflammation**
Skin Repair	Top choice for scars, moisture, elasticity	Good, but not its strongest area
Hormonal Support	Strong support for fertility, PMS, menopause	Moderate
Antioxidant Power	Strong	**Extremely strong — tocotrienols act faster**
Unique Nutrients	Octacosanol (endurance, energy)	**Carotenoids (pro-vitamin A), CoQ10-like compounds**

Benefit Category	*Wheat Germ Oil*	*Red Palm Oil*
Anti-Cancer Research	Limited	Emerging research shows tocotrienols may slow tumor growth
Cooking Stability	Not stable—use as a supplement	Very stable for low–medium heat cooking

3. How They Differ in the Body

Wheat Germ Oil

- Rebuilds and moisturizes skin deeply
- Supports reproductive health and hormonal rhythm
- Nourishes the liver
- Boosts oxygen flow to tissues
- Promotes wound healing

Red Palm Oil

- Feeds the **brain**, especially when paired with iodine + selenium
- Reduces inflammation at the cellular level
- Protects neurons from oxidative damage
- Strengthens the cardiovascular system
- Delivers massive amounts of **beta-carotene + vitamin A**

4. When to Use Which?

Choose Wheat Germ Oil if you want:

- Skin healing
- Fertility support
- Hair growth
- Hormonal balance
- Gentle, daily antioxidant protection

Choose Red Palm Oil if you want:

- Brain protection
- Child development support
- Strong antioxidant therapy
- Cardiovascular protection
- Vitamin A + tocotrienols for deep cellular repair

Best practice:
Use both — they complete each other.
Together, they form the full spectrum of Vitamin E the body actually needs.
Wheat germ oil feeds the body.
Red palm oil feeds the brain.
Together, they restore the whole person.

Health is not complicated when we remember the wisdom of nature. Our suffering begins when we forget Mother Nature's design.

Iodine, selenium, and Vitamin E are not luxuries. They are part of the original blueprint.

CHAPTER 24 BIBLIOGRAPHY

1. **Kohrle, Josef.** "Thyroid Hormones, Selenium, and Functional Hypothyroidism: A Review." *Biological Trace Element Research*, 2025. https://link.springer.com/article/10.1007/s12011-025-04653-7.
2. **Zimmermann, Michael B.** "Iodine Deficiency." *Endocrine Reviews* 30, no. 4 (2009): 376–408. https://doi.org/10.1210/er.2009-0011.
(A gold-standard scientific review on iodine's role in human biology, deficiency, thyroid function, pregnancy, and brain development.)
3. **Salonen, J. T., et al.** "Effect of Vitamin E and Selenium on Atherosclerosis in Mice." *Circulation Research* 83, no. 4 (1998): 366–372. https://www.ahajournals.org/doi/10.1161/01.res.83.4.366.

CHAPTER 25

BRILLIANT FOREVER

*Intelligence is not something you lose with age—
it is something you preserve with wisdom.*

Have you ever sat with an elder who remembers whole lifetime, who names the past the way someone names the rooms in their home? Their memory glows. Their stories steady you. Their presence makes children bolder and families wiser.

Communities in Okinawa still hold this gift—neighborhoods guided by elders who live past one hundred and still teach, laugh, and lead. That is what was taken from us: not just long life, but the wisdom-keepers who were meant to guide our children. And this is exactly what we are reclaiming—**our longevity, our brilliance, our elders.**

Life begins and ends with the health of the brain.

Memory loss, dementia, Alzheimer's disease, diabetes, and mental decline are **not** natural parts of aging. They are signs of imbalance—missing nutrients, inflammation, and forgotten ancestral knowledge.

Sage for Memory

Sage has been used for centuries to "strengthen the brain and the memory." Research now confirms it. Sage sharpens recall, improves focus, and protects the brain by supporting acetylcholine—the chemical of learning—while reducing inflammation and oxidative stress.

Boswellia (Frankincense): Wisdom from the Ancients

Thee healing power of **Boswellia**. Our ancestors treasured it for calming inflammation, sharpening memory, and protecting the mind.

One of the Three Wise Men offered frankincense to the Christ child—not as decoration, but as medicine, protection and spiritual wisdom.

"This section is dedicated to my big brother, Rofe Malakael, a healer, for his wisdom and inspiration regarding Boswellia."

Modern research now confirms its gifts - Boswellia:

- supports healthy blood sugar
- reduces inflammation and pain
- protects brain cells
- improves short-term memory
- strengthens immunity
- supports gut healing
- promotes healthy cholesterol

Does Boswellia Help with Strokes?

Yes—indirectly and significantly. Boswellia:

- protects brain cells from dying
- reduces the inflammation that worsens stroke damage
- supports blood vessel healing
- improves cognitive recovery
- Boswellia guards the mind.

The Power of Millet

It's time to let the rice, wheat and corn go as often as possible! Millet is more than a food — it is a medicinal grain with the power to restore and protect the body. Research shows that regular millet consumption can lower the risk of heart disease, improve blood sugar control, strengthen digestion, reduce cancer risk, and support detoxification pathways.

Millet also boosts respiratory immunity, raises energy levels, and nourishes both the muscular and nervous systems. Its antioxidant-rich profile offers protection against age-related degenerative conditions, including metabolic syndrome and Parkinson's disease (Manach et al., 2005; Scalbert et al., 2005).

In short: millet is not just nourishment — it is prevention, resilience, and longevity on a plate.

Below is a concise, polished summary of the benefits of FIVE key millets:

Barnyard Millet — The Blood Sugar & Heart Protector

Barnyard millet consistently shows the **strongest ability to lower blood glucose, cholesterol, and triglycerides** compared with rice and other millets (Kumari & Thayumanavan, 1997).

Its **low glycemic index** (41.7–50.0) makes it ideal for type 2 diabetes (Ugare et al., 2011).

It is rich in fiber, minerals, and antioxidants that support:

- Heart health
- Steady energy
- Weight management
- Reduced inflammation
- Lower risk of cardiovascular complications

Barnyard millet is one of the most powerful "everyday medicines" in the grain world.

Foxtail Millet — Anti-Diabetic & Anti-Inflammatory

Foxtail millet contains compounds that have shown **excellent anti-hyperglycemic activity** (Sireesha et al., 2011).

It supports:

- Blood sugar control
- Lower inflammation
- Improved metabolic health

Its antioxidants also help protect the nervous system and reduce oxidative stress.

Proso Millet — Insulin Support & Cancer Protection

Proso millet improves **glycemic response and insulin levels** even in genetically obese type 2 diabetic models (Park et al., 2008).

Research links the fiber and phytochemicals in sorghum and millets (including proso millet) to:

- Lower risk of colon and breast cancer
- Lower risk of esophageal cancer (Graf & Eaton, 1990; Van Rensburg, 1981)
- Proso millet is a metabolic and cellular protector.

Finger Millet — The Cardiovascular Shield

Finger millet significantly lowers **serum triglycerides** compared to white rice and sorghum (Lee et al., 2010).

It is also naturally rich in:

- Calcium
- Iron
- Fiber
- Antioxidants

This makes it excellent for:

- Bone health (especially for women)
- Hormonal balance
- Heart protection
- Lowering inflammation

Finger millet is a heart-loving, hormone-supporting grain.

Kodo Millet — Postmenopausal Protector & Mineral Powerhouse

Kodo millet is rich in **B vitamins (B6, niacin, folate)** and minerals like calcium, iron, magnesium, potassium, and zinc. It is **gluten-free** and especially beneficial for:

- Postmenopausal women (lowering blood pressure and cholesterol)
- Cardiovascular health
- Hormonal stability
- Nervous system strength

Kodo millet offers remarkable support where women need it most.

When glucose is stable and the cardiovascular system is strong, the brain can think faster, age slower, and preserve intelligence across decades.

This is not just longevity — this is **brilliance preserved**.

Why Deficiency Creeps In

Deficiencies appear not because the body forgets—but because *we* forget. Life gets busy. Meals lose minerals. Supplements are skipped. Stress rises. And slowly, silently, the brain and body weaken.

Intelligence isn't lost—it is unsupported.
Memory doesn't fade—it is unfed.
Longevity isn't gone—it is waiting.

Put herbs and minerals back on the plate and let the earth and sea guard your brilliance for life.

CHAPTER 25 BIBLIOGRAPHY

SAGE (COGNITION & MEMORY)

1. **Akhondzadeh, S., et al.** "Salvia officinalis Extract in the Treatment of Patients with Mild to Moderate Alzheimer's Disease: A Double-Blind, Randomized and Placebo-Controlled Trial." *Journal of Clinical Pharmacy and Therapeutics* 28, no. 1 (2003): 53–59.
2. **Tildesley, N. T. J., et al.** "Salvia (Sage) Effects on Cognition and Mood in Healthy Adults." *Pharmacology, Biochemistry and Behavior* 75, no. 3 (2003): 669–674.

BOSWELLIA / FRANKINCENSE
(BRAIN, INFLAMMATION, STROKES, MEMORY)

3. **Hosseini-Sharifabad, M., and M. E. Esfandiary.** "Effect of Boswellia serrata Resin on Spatial Learning and Memory in Rats." *Journal of Ethnopharmacology* 102, no. 2 (2005): 215–219.
4. **Siddiqui, M. Z.** "Boswellia serrata: A Potential Antiinflammatory Agent." *Indian Journal of Pharmaceutical Sciences* 73, no. 3 (2011): 255–261.
5. **Gerbeth, K., et al.** "Boswellic Acids Reduce Neuroinflammation and Improve Cognitive Function." *Phytomedicine* 19, no. 12 (2012): 1043–1050.

MILLET (BLOOD SUGAR, HEART, METABOLISM, ANTIOXIDANTS, POSTMENOPAUSAL HEALTH)
General Millet Antioxidant Sources:

6. **Manach, C., et al.** "Polyphenols: Food Sources and Bioavailability." *American Journal of Clinical Nutrition* 79, no. 5 (2004): 727–747.
7. **Scalbert, A., et al.** "Polyphenols and the Prevention of Diseases." *Critical Reviews in Food Science and Nutrition* 45, no. 4 (2005): 287–306.

Barnyard Millet

8. **Kumari, P. L., and B. Thayumanavan.** "Barnyard Millet in Diabetes Control." *Journal of Food Science and Technology* 34, no. 4 (1997): 316–319.
9. **Ugare, R., et al.** "Glycemic Index of Barnyard Millet." *Journal of Food Science and Technology* 48, no. 4 (2011): 591–594.

Foxtail Millet

10. **Sireesha, K., et al.** "Anti-Hyperglycemic Effects of Foxtail Millet." *International Journal of Diabetes in Developing Countries* 31, no. 3 (2011): 140–146.

Proso Millet

11. **Park, J. H., et al.** "Proso Millet Improves Insulin Sensitivity in Type 2 Diabetes." *Nutrition Research and Practice* 2, no. 3 (2008): 152–158.
12. **Graf, E., and J. W. Eaton.** "Antioxidants in Cereal Grain Fiber." *Journal of Nutrition* 120, no. 1 (1990): 52–58.
13. **Van Rensburg, S. J.** "Epidemiologic Evidence for Sorghum and Millet in Cancer Prevention." *Nutritional Cancer* 3, no. 2 (1981): 93–98.

Finger Millet

14. **Lee, S. H., et al.** "Finger Millet Lowers Lipids and Triglycerides." *Nutrition Research* 30, no. 6 (2010): 414–419.

Kodo Millet

15. **Chandrasekara, A., and Fereidoon Shahidi.** "Bioactive Compounds in Millet and Postmenopausal Health." *Journal of Functional Foods* 5, no. 1 (2013): 470–485.

LONGEVITY / OKINAWA

16. **Willcox, Bradley J., D. Craig Willcox, and Makoto Suzuki.** *The Okinawa Program: How the World's Longest-Lived People Achieve Everlasting Health.* New York: Clarkson Potter, 2001.

CHAPTER 26

NOURISH YOUR DESTINY

Science can fill pages, but stories touch the heart. While research and data prove the role of iodine, selenium, red palm oil, and cod liver oil in building intelligence and resilience, the most powerful evidence comes from the lives of people who lived it. These testimonies are not theories. They are **living proof** that nourishment changes destinies. The following are testimonies of my close friends between 60 and 80 years old.

Mr. E.O. – Nigeria

My dear friend, Mr. E.O., grew up in Nigeria—a nation that actively embraced the iodized salt program. As a boy, every Sunday meant a faithful spoonful of cod liver oil. His diet was rich with red palm oil, and his family enjoyed fresh cod and mackerel straight from the ocean.

That foundation carried him into adulthood, where he became a scholar and educator in physics, chemistry, and advanced mathematics. He credits not only his studies but also his spirituality, clean living, and the wisdom of health practices passed down by his parents and ancestors.

Now in his seventies, Mr. E.O. lives with the vitality of a teenager:

- For the past decades, he has maintained a strict vegan diet.
- He takes no medications.
- His immune system is strong and steady.
- He rides his bicycle for long stretches with ease.
- His thinking remains sharp; his memory is amazingly clear.
- His vision is still 20/20—so he does not require prescription or reading glasses.

When he read my work, Mr. E.O. said, *"Thank you, for your research on minerals. Your work is impressive, and it confirms what I have lived."* His story is a witness that consistent nourishment, paired with faith and discipline, preserves the mind and body for a lifetime.

Michelle R. – Westland, Michigan

Michelle R. and I have been friends since the eighth grade, and unlike so many others, she **never stopped taking cod liver oil.** The results spoke for themselves.

As a child, Michelle was unstoppable:

- Her grades were exceptional.
- She typed 90 words per minute when most of us struggled to reach 60 words because it was not about how fast our fingers moved but about how fast the brain could process.
- Michelle was a champion athlete, winning in track and field.
- Her vocabulary and mastery of English were far beyond her peers.
- Her hair still today is long, thick, and radiant—a crown of health.

As a mother and grandmother, the blessings multiplied:

- She experienced uncomplicated pregnancies and natural births.
- Her children and grandchildren grew strong, healthy, and advanced. Her daughter Shekaiya's testimony is in Stolen Intellect I.

Michelle continues to astonish her supervisors. They say she works at the pace of three people, processing information with remarkable speed and clarity. This is not luck — it is the result of lifelong nourishment. Michelle is living proof that health, intelligence, and minerals compound across generations.

Clara F. – Ann Arbor, Michigan

Clara's grandmother was faithful: every single day from childhood until high school graduation, Clara received her spoonful of cod liver oil. The results shaped her destiny.

- She excelled academically and was consistently placed in honors classes.
- She earned a college scholarship.

- She majored in engineering, thriving in advanced mathematics.
- She rose in the finance world, eventually becoming a regional manager overseeing eight banks.

Now in her early 60s, Clara admits she didn't always connect her success to cod liver oil. But looking back, she sees how its daily nourishment sharpened her mind, fueled her energy, and gave her the stamina to lead with confidence. Her story is a reminder that small, faithful habits create legacies of strength.

Robert J. – California

Robert's story is different—and powerful. He grew up swimming in the ocean almost daily and vividly remember taking cod liver oil regularly as a child.

In elementary school, Robert thrived under enthusiastic teachers. But by middle school, things shifted. Teachers grew timid, fearful of their students, and Robert lost interest. By high school, he walked away from formal education altogether.

Yet Robert's intelligence was undeniable. His creativity, sharp mind, and tireless work ethic led him to entrepreneurship. As a single father, he built a thriving company—and more importantly, he hired his own children. He paid them wages, taught them banking skills, and showed them how to endorse, deposit their check, and pay a bill at a very young age.

Later, Robert earned his GED. Today, he is a proud grandfather, surrounded by adult children who are financially stable, responsible, and successful.

Robert's life is proof that true intelligence is not measured by diplomas. It comes from a nourished brain, a strong spirit, and the wisdom to pass knowledge on. His story reminds us that when nutrition and values meet, generational wealth and stability follow.

Reflection: Testimonies for Teaching

These stories are not fairy tales. They are the lived experiences of men and women whose lives were nourished with cod liver oil, iodine, and minerals from the ocean. They remind us that intelligence, health, and resilience are not accidents of birth; they are the fruit of nourishment.

Mr. E.O.'s life is proof that when a nation embraces iodized salt, cod liver oil, and traditional foods like red palm oil, entire generations can thrive with clarity, strength, and vitality into their seventies and beyond. Michelle shows us the blessing of lifelong faithfulness to nourishment. Clara demonstrates how a grandmother's daily care can shape a granddaughter's future in academics and leadership. Robert reveals that even when education is interrupted, a nourished brain and strong spirit can build businesses, raise healthy and wise children, and create financial stability.

Together, these lives remind us that the daily nourishment is the seed of generational brilliance. Whether carried through cultural traditions, sustained by faithful family habits, or strengthened by personal discipline, the root cause remains the same: wherever minerals are honored, health, genius and sound mind flourish.

A Lesson from the Movie -Avatar

Stories of nourishment are not limited to real life. Even movies like *Avatar* hold hidden truths.

In the film, the Tree People were resilient warriors, but when their world was attacked, they had to flee to where the Ocean People lived. When the Tree People arrived, they were astonished: the Ocean People were taller, stronger, more colorful, faster, and more intelligent.

The longer the Tree People lived by the ocean, the sharper they became. They learned to swim with speed, to breathe underwater, and to adapt in ways that expanded their intelligence and capacity.

The message is clear: **the ocean is the ultimate nourishment.** It unites all the elements—sea, air, sun, earth, moon, and stars—into one powerful symphony of life.

Final Word

We must never forget education begins with nourishment. Without it, no diploma or degree can replace what the body and brain lack. With it, people can live, learn, lead, and thrive far beyond what we have imagined.

CHAPTER 27

THE DARKNESS WE INHERITED

"Darkness covered the earth, and gross darkness (ignorance) covered the people."

This scripture was never meant to describe our destiny, only our condition. *But no one said we had to remain in the darkness either.* Revelation declares, "Satan deceived **the whole world**."

So, the question becomes unavoidable:

Who deceived us? Who dimmed our brilliance? Who stole our minerals?

Not an enemy far away.

Not a stranger in the shadows.

Deception comes from those close enough to shape what we believe, teach what we accept, and silence what we question.

1. Who Deceived Us?

The Ones Standing Closest

I was taught, "Keep your friends close, but your enemies closer."

Who is close enough to mislead a nation?

Who occupies the inner circles of trust? Who sits on panels, writes policies, and shapes the way we think? Who is close enough to teach us what not to see? Close enough to normalize deficiency as disease?

As I awakened to ancient memories, I began to see the blueprint: Institutions were not separate parts—they were synchronized instruments, moving in lockstep, gatekeeping the truth about minerals, nutrition, human intelligence, religion and education.

2. Education: The Rockefeller Way

If you fund the lesson plan, you shape the lessons.
If you shape the lessons, you shape the mind.
If you shape the mind, you shape the nation.
American institutions trained us to trust—not question.

A Personal Story

A year ago, a midwifery student overheard my conversation about the necessity of iodine for mothers and toddlers.

She said aloud, with complete conviction:

"Your theory doesn't exist."

I was stunned. Offended. But with clarity, I realized:

She wasn't being cruel—**she was repeating the ignorance she had been taught.**

This is why debates with clinicians feel circular.

Why truth feels foreign.

Why prevention feels "controversial."

The system teaches clinicians what to notice and what to ignore. Deficiencies disappear under mountains of disease labels. And the mineral model—the real root-cause model—is dismissed before the first lecture begins.

3. The Death Certificate That Lies

No coroner writes:

- *"Died from lack of iodine."*
- *"Died from a lack of selenium."*
- *"Died from vitamin C deficiency."*
- *"Died from vitamin E deficiency*
- *"Died from iron deficiency"*
- *"Died from vitamin D deficiency"*
- *"Died from potassium deficiency"*
- *"Died from magnesium deficiency"*

Instead, they write: **"Death by Natural Causes."** As if death is natural when the body has been starved of nutrients vital for survival. Behind the scenes of gross darkness is…..

Death by ocean deficiency, Death by sun deficiency.

All this time, the real truth is these are just deficiencies masquerading as mysterious diseases.

We do not die of disease.
We die of depletion.
We die of gaps.
We die of missing elements from the firmament.

4. When Homes Were Healing Centers

A matriarchal society is a social system in which women—particularly mothers and elder women—serve as cultural anchors, guiding family continuity, caregiving, moral education, and the transmission of values across generations. Authority is rooted not in domination, but in nurturance, wisdom, and responsibility for collective well-being.

In healthy matriarchal systems, men are not displaced; they are essential partners—protectors, builders, teachers, and stewards—whose leadership complements maternal guidance. Decision-making is shared, lineage is preserved, and community stability is prioritized through cooperation rather than hierarchy.

At its best, a matriarchal society is family-centered, life-protecting, and future-oriented, ensuring that children, elders, and men alike are supported so the entire community thrives.

Our mothers and grandmothers were the healers.

- Seaweed in the pot
- Cod liver oil on the spoon
- Red palm oil in the pan
- Herbs on the shelf
- Bone broths for strength
- Sunlight for immunity
- Warmth, wisdom, and watchfulness

These women safeguarded their families with elemental knowledge. Today, we rush to urgent care for what used to be treated in the kitchen.

And when labs are drawn?

The very minerals that matter most are rarely measured: Institutions don't check for what you need daily: iodine, vitamin A, vitamin E, vitamin C, zinc or selenium. They are your front-line defense team.

This isn't nostalgia. This is a call to restore a broken covenant between home and ancient healing wisdom.

5. We Are MinerallyMade — Not Disease-Made:

We were formed from the dust of the earth, the minerals of the sea, and the light of the sun.

NHANES Data Tells the Story (16,444 participants ages 4 years old and up). These are not diseases, but death by natural causes if we don't supplement.

Nutrient	% Below Needs	Reality Check
Vitamin D	94.3% below	Almost the whole nation deficient
Vitamin E	88.5% below	One of the sharpest deficiencies
Magnesium	52.2% below	Over half below need
Calcium	44.1% below	Nearly half deficient
Vitamin A	43% below	Persistent deficiency
Vitamin C	38.9% below	One-third deficient
Potassium	100% below	A heart attack waiting to happen.
Choline	91.7% below	Essential for brain development
Vitamin K	66.9% below	Two-thirds below AI
Sodium	97% above UL	Too much processed food

Note: Adequate Intake (**AI**)
Upper Limit (**UL**)

6. The Silent Collapse of Women

Women lose the most minerals:

- Each menstrual cycle
- Each trimester of pregnancy
- Each birth
- Each period of stress
- Each round of environmental toxins

Iron needs rise from 18 mg to 27 mg in pregnancy, yet **70% of deficiencies go undiagnosed** (Weyand et al., 2023).

This is biological sabotage disguised as "routine care."

7. The Gift of the Ocean: Seaweed as Salvation

Seaweed: Vitamins & Minerals at a Glance

So here is a gentle reminder: there is an easy, beautiful way to weave minerals and vitamins into your daily rhythm, without stress and without making it complicated.

Firmament foods! Where the sea meets the earth

Seaweed	Vitamins	Minerals
Nori (Porphyra/Pyropia)	A (carotenoids), C, K, B1, B2, B3, B6; B12 (reported)	Iodine, Iron, Calcium, Magnesium, Potassium, Copper, Manganese, Zinc,
Wakame (Undaria)	A, C, E, K, Folate (B9), B2	Iodine, Iron, Calcium, Magnesium, Potassium, Copper, Manganese, Phosphorus,
Kombu/Kelp (Laminaria)	A, C, B1, B2, B6	Very high -Iodine; Iron, Calcium, Magnesium, Potassium; Selenium (trace)
Dulse (Palmaria)	A (carotenoids), C, B-vitamins; E	Iodine, Iron, Calcium, Magnesium, Potassium, Zinc, Manganese
Sea Lettuce (Ulva)	C, A, K, B-vitamins (reports include B12)	Iodine, Iron, Calcium, Magnesium, Potassium, Zinc
Irish Moss / "Sea Moss" (Chondrus)	Folate (B9), other B vitamins; antioxidants	Iodine, Iron, Calcium, Magnesium, Potassium, Zinc
Arame (Eisenia)	A, K, some B vitamins	Iodine, Iron, Calcium, Magnesium, Potassium, trace elements
Bladderwrack (Fucus)	A, C, E; B-vitamins	Iodine, Iron, Calcium, Magnesium, Potassium, Selenium (trace)
Hijiki (Hizikia/Sargassum)	A, K; some B vitamins	Iodine, Iron, Calcium, Magnesium, Potassium

Minerallymade, LLC For educational purposes only

Seaweed is not just food;
It is elemental memory.
It is intelligence restored.
It is the ocean on your plate.

Animals instinctively move toward mineral-rich shores when their bodies need replenishment. Humans once followed the same pattern — until we were indoctrinated to forget.

8. A Call to Wisdom

To every parent, grandparent, and elder:
You are sacred. You are essential. And your life holds immeasurable value.

- Take your minerals.
- Restore your strength.
- Bring back the sea into your body.
- Reclaim the sunlight that built your cells.
- Return to the elements that built the mind.

The ocean has never stopped offering its gifts — reach for them.

9. The Gift of Presence

When our minds are nourished and our bodies are strong, we naturally turn toward our purpose instead of pain, discomfort, illness, or limitation. My prayer for you — as you read these pages — is that you rediscover ancient healing wisdom that helps you return your attention to why you came here, to the true reason you exist.

Your children, grandchildren, great-grandchildren, and great-great-grandchildren need you *alive, wise and well.*

Your **wisdom is medicine.**
Your **longevity is protection.**
Your **presence is irreplaceable.**
We need you.

CHAPTER 27 BIBLIOGRAPHY

1. **Wallace, Taylor C., Michael McBurney, and Victor L. Fulgoni III.**
   "Multivitamin/Mineral Supplement Contribution to Micronutrient Intakes in the United States, 2007–2010."
   Journal of the American College of Nutrition 33, no. 2 (2014): 94–102.

2. **Weyand, A. C., et al.**
   "Prevalence of Iron Deficiency and Iron-Deficiency Anemia in US Females Aged 12–21 Years, 2003–2020."
   JAMA 329, no. 24 (2023): 2191–2193.

3. **Rayman, Margaret P.**
   "The Importance of Selenium to Human Health."
   The Lancet 356, no. 9225 (2000): 233–241.

4. **Zimmermann, Michael B.**
   "Iodine Deficiency."
   Endocrine Reviews 30, no. 4 (2009): 376–408.

5. **Holick, Michael F.**
   "Vitamin D Deficiency."
   New England Journal of Medicine 357 (2007): 266–281.

6. **Mouritsen, Ole G., et al.**
   "Seaweeds for Umami and Nutrition."
   Flavour 2, no. 17 (2013).

7. **Ames, Bruce N.**
   "A Role for Micronutrient Deficiency in Aging: Triage Theory."
   Proceedings of the National Academy of Sciences 103, no. 47 (2006): 17589–17594.

8. **Price, Weston A.**
   Nutrition and Physical Degeneration. Paul B. Hoeber, 1939.

CHAPTER 28

IODINE: THE FORGOTTEN FIRST AID

All throughout this book, I refer to minerals like **J. Crow's Lugol's Iodine**—a lot! And for good reasons. You should always have it on hand, so don't hesitate to use it. When emergencies strike—a cut, scrape, bite, burn, or sudden skin flare—your first line of defense doesn't need to be an antibiotic ointment.

Long before modern medicine, iodine was the world's most trusted topical antiseptic—used in homes, hospitals, clinics, and military field kits. It still works. Iodine rapidly inactivates bacteria, viruses, fungi, and even some parasites **on contact**, giving the wound a chance to heal cleanly and preventing infection in minor injuries.

In a world where we reach for pharmaceuticals first, it's important to remember:

Some of the most powerful tools for healing were here long before antibiotics—and iodine is one of them.

When to Reach for Iodine

- **Dirty cuts & scrapes** – disinfect before infection takes hold.
- **Dog bite, animal bite, spider bites** – use iodine to kill as many invading organisms as possible before they enter the wound.
- **Insect stings, mosquito & tick bites** – Remove the stinger if possible, then add iodine.
- **Nail salon germs** – If you feel a microscopic itch, or infection after pedicures or manicures, seek medical advice if you need to but add iodine to kill any invading organisms before they cause severe damage.
- **Dark moles or keloid scars** – support natural skin repair.
- **Pre-cancerous lumps, skin tags or odd skin lesions** – Apply iodine to encourage healthy cell turnover.
- **Everyday scratches & abrasions** – quick, safe protection for kids and adults.

A few drops or swabs of iodine on a small cut or scrape may help lower the chance of infection and sometimes prevent problems that could otherwise send you to the emergency room —serious wounds don't hesitate to seek medical care.

CHAPTER 28 BIBLIOGRAPHY

1. **Weston A. Price Foundation.** "The Great Iodine Debate."
   Weston A. Price Foundation. https://www.westonaprice.org.
2. **Morell, Geoffrey, N.D.** Case reports on iodine therapy, as summarized in "The Great Iodine Debate," Weston A. Price Foundation.
3. **Derry, David.** Commentary on apoptosis and topical iodine for skin healing, as quoted in "The Great Iodine Debate," Weston A. Price Foundation.

"When you teach a woman,
you teach a nation"

CHAPTER 29

MOTHERS WIT

We once relied on **Mothers' Wit—mothers' wisdom.** Doctors were *not* the first line of defense when I was growing up, our mothers and grandmothers were there! They carried with them generations of inherited wisdom, remedies born from observation, prayer, and Divine Intelligence.

When I became a mother, I still leaned on that lineage. Every time one of my children was sick, I picked up the phone to call my mom or my grandmother, because I knew they would know what to do. And just as they poured into me, I found myself becoming a healer and pouring into people too. What I do know is this:

Mother Nature has never been confused about healing — we have.

Every answer we search for in hospitals and laboratories first existed in the ocean, in the soil, in the sunlight, and in the foods our ancestors trusted.

My mantra for all mothers is this:

Disease is not real. Deficiency is.

Disease creates fear.

Deficiency creates understanding.

Disease blames the body.

Deficiency teaches us what the body needs.

Disease makes us feel powerless.

Deficiency empowers us to prevent what others call "inevitable."

When we shift our thinking from disease to deficiency, everything changes:

Instead of asking, *"What is wrong with me?"*

we begin asking, *"What is missing from me?"*

And that question leads us back to the firmament — the minerals of the sea, the vitamins of the sun, the gifts of the earth.

A Mouth Full of Fever Blisters

I will never forget when my son was four years old. The inside of his mouth—cheeks, tongue, and palate—was covered in blisters. We were out of the country at the time, but I didn't panic. I picked up the phone and called my grandmother, Pearl, in Detroit.

She didn't hesitate. First, he had a fever, so those are fever-blisters in his mouth. Clean his colon out with a mild laxative," she said. I did exactly as she instructed, and within no time, my son was back to normal. That day I realized something powerful: fevers, blisters, and sickness weren't mysteries to my grandmother. She understood the order of symptoms and the remedies to restore balance. Her wisdom was sharper than any medical textbook.

Protecting the Daughters Who Carry Tomorrow

Our daughters are born with all the eggs they will ever have — a complete library of future generations already inside their tiny bodies. From the moment a baby girl enters the world, she is not just one life; she is **many lives waiting in silence**, carried in her ovaries like seeds waiting for the right season.

And that means something profound:

When we protect our daughters, we are protecting our grandchildren and great-grandchildren.

When we neglect our daughters, we injure generations we will never meet.

A girl's eggs are formed in the womb, nourished — or weakened — by her mother's mineral status, her mother's environment, and her mother's exposure to toxins. By the time a girl is born, the quality of her eggs has already been shaped by:

- iodine levels
- selenium status
- Vitamin A and D
- exposure to perchlorates (rocket fuel)
- pollution and highway toxins
- microplastics, smoke, and endocrine disruptors
- stress, poor nutrition, and mineral depletion

Those eggs remain with her through childhood, adolescence, womanhood, and motherhood. They age with her, suffer with her, strengthen with her. Every toxin she encounters — fireworks smoke, highway exhaust, contaminated water, heavy metals — touches not just her body, but the eggs she carries.

And every nutrient she receives — iodine, selenium, cod liver oil, iron, red palm oil, seaweed — nourishes her future babies before she herself becomes a mother.

This is why iodine is not optional.

This is why minerals are not optional.

This is why protection must begin early — long before pregnancy.

A mother and father's first responsibility is not only to the child they raise, but to the children that child will one day carry.

Fathers protect the family by making sure the home is fed with iodine-rich foods and clean minerals.

Mothers protect the lineage by nourishing their own bodies and shielding their daughters from toxic environments.

Every choice today becomes biology tomorrow.

Every nutrient today becomes intelligence tomorrow.

Every protection today becomes a legacy tomorrow.

When we protect our daughters' eggs:

- We protect fertility
- We protect IQ
- We protect emotional stability
- We protect thyroid and hormonal balance
- We protect the next generation's health, wisdom, and strength

A girl is not just somebody's daughter.
She is **the keeper of a nation's future.**
She carries the possibility of generations the world has not yet seen.

And that is why mothers and fathers must rise now — with awareness, with intention, with iodine, with truth — because the choices we make today will echo into the next hundred years.

Your eggs formed long before you were born. When you nourish yourself, you also nourish the generations inside you. Minerals feed your fertility, your future children, and their children.

Toxic Exposures

- Living near busy highways exposes the womb and a baby's developing brain to exhaust pollutants.
- Fireworks release heavy metals and toxins that can damage the eggs inside our daughters long before they ever conceive.

These exposures are modern forms of chemical sabotage — silent, invisible, and completely preventable. And standing between these toxins and your unborn child is one mineral: **iodine**.

Iodine fortifies the thyroid, shields the fetus, and protects the eggs of our daughters from many of these environmental assaults.

Without iodine, these toxins strike harder.

With iodine, the body has its natural armor.

A Cancer Story: Healing Against the Odds

Mother Nature has the wisdom and the answers for everything health. Here is an example:

One day at a baby shower, a tall, handsome young man with a glowing complexion sat beside me and said, **"Thank you."** I didn't recognize him, but he reminded me that four months earlier I had sent Lugol's iodine and selenium (selenium excell brand) to his sister—for him.

At that time, he was thirty years old and gravely ill with cancer. His family had already gathered at the hospital fearing the worst. He had been bleeding from his eyes and other orifices, losing weight rapidly, and growing weaker despite cancer medications.

But that night the supplements arrived; he stated that he stopped taking his cancer medication and took the supplements instead. The morning after he began taking the two supplements, he woke up with unexpected energy. "Momma, I feel good today!" he told his mother.

He continued taking them daily, and over the next several months he regained weight, strength, and life. During the baby shower, he told me something else:

"For the first four months, my doctors assumed I was still taking the cancer medication. I never told them I stopped and switched to supplements."

The young man stated that he kept every doctor's appointment, and his physician team marveled at how well he was doing.

Now, there I was looking up at him for the first time. He was standing tall, vibrant, and full of color. About 6 feet tall, a nice full afro and his weight – the epitome of health. No one would have guessed he had once been at death's door.

Next, I said to him, "Now that you are well, please don't buy a new car." Quickly, he said, "I already bought one and my face swelled immediately afterwards, so, I called my doctors, and they asked, "was there anything new that you ate or were exposed to?" He said, "not that I can think of."

Interestingly, when I share this story with others, they always ask the same question , "Why did you suggest he not buy a new car?"

I already knew a new car could compromise his weak immune system. That sharp "new car smell" comes from **chemicals slowly releasing (off-gassing)** from the car's interior—especially when the car is warm.

What You Should Know About Your "New Car Smell"

Where does it come from? The main sources are:

- **Seat foam** (often treated with flame retardants)
- **Carpets and floor padding**
- **Dashboards and door panels**
- **Ceiling fabric (headliner)**
- **Glues and adhesives**

These materials release **volatile organic compounds (VOCs)** into the air. Some of the same materials also contain **bromine-based flame retardants**, which can interfere with hormone and thyroid signaling over time.

Why Children Are Also More Vulnerable

- Children breathe **more air per pound of body weight**
- Their brains and hormones are **still developing**
- They often sit closer to seats and surfaces that release chemicals
- Heat increases exposure (parked cars can exceed 140°F)

This doesn't mean panic—it means *awareness and simple protection.*

Simple Ways Parents Can Reduce Exposure

- **Ventilate new cars** (open doors/windows before driving)
- **Avoid sitting in hot, parked cars**
- **Use fresh air instead of recirculated air**
- **Park in shade or garages when possible**
- **Vacuum regularly** to reduce chemical dust
- **Wash hands after long car rides**, especially before eating

Nutrition Matters Too

The body's ability to handle environmental exposure depends on **nutritional protection**.

Adequate levels of:

- **Iodine**
- **Selenium**
- **Iron**
- **Calcium**
- **Vitamin C**

help support the body's natural defense and detoxification systems. Modern safety standards protect cars from fire but nutrition protects children from chemical overload.

CHAPTER 29 BIBLIOGRAPHY

1. **Environmental Working Group (EWG).** "Colorado River Contamination: Perchlorate in Produce." Environmental Working Group.
2. **National Research Council (NRC).** *Health Implications of Perchlorate Ingestion.* Washington, DC: National Academies Press, 2005.
3. **U.S. Food and Drug Administration (FDA)** and **U.S. Environmental Protection Agency (EPA).** Reports on perchlorate contamination in leafy greens and irrigation water.

4. **Bergman, Åke, et al.** *State of the Science on Endocrine Disrupting Chemicals.* World Health Organization and United Nations Environment Programme, 2013.

5. **Block, Michelle L., and Lilian Calderón-Garcidueñas.** "Air Pollution: Mechanisms of Neuroinflammation and Neurodegeneration." *Trends in Neurosciences* 35, no. 9 (2012): 506–516.

6. **Clemente, D.B.P., et al.** "Prenatal Exposure to Air Pollution and Child Neurodevelopment." *Environmental Health Perspectives* 128, no. 6 (2020).

7. **Jha, A.K., et al.** "Pollution from Fireworks: Metal Contamination and Health Effects." *Environmental Monitoring and Assessment* 189, no. 10 (2017).

8. **U.S. Environmental Protection Agency (EPA).** Reports on particulate emissions and heavy metals released by fireworks.

CHAPTER 30

B.B.I.B.L.E.

(Basic Breast care Instructions Before Leaving Earth)

Healthy breasts are not a miracle or a mystery—they are your birthright.
This chapter belongs to our daughters, our teens, our sisters, our mothers—every woman in every season of life.

You Were Crafted from Creation

Daughters of the Divine—you are so remarkable that the Creator placed a special diet in creation just for you. You were made from the elements of the earth, the seas and the sun. The same miracles written across the firmament are written in you. But minerals deplete, and it becomes your sacred responsibility to restore them.

When you crave food, your body is not asking for "anything"—it is calling for what you were made from. Your brain, breasts, and womb remember the sea. That is why they ask for sea gifts: seaweed, iodine-rich foods, and selenium.

When you were born you brought with you all your eggs too. So, you are not nourishing only yourself—you are also nourishing the **eggs within you**, any of them have the potential to fertilize and will one day be the **child you carry**. These same minerals you need, the eggs inside you need them too.

These gifts are part of a sacred covenant between you and the Divine. The Divine Feminine was never meant to be cut off from Mother Nature; Disconnections mean imbalances can appear— breast tenderness, cysts, and other breasts and womb troubles.

The rays of the sun, the pull of the moon, the oceans, and the earth all echo inside you. In them are the minerals and vitamins for your hormone health—**a perfect cosmic recipe** so generous we were never meant to be without them.

Breast-Care Wisdom Was Always in You

If we lived in a true matriarchal society (societies that highly respect, honor and value women), you would have already known how to protect your breasts and womb at an early age.

Studies show breasts tissue *stores* iodine, especially during pregnancy and lactation. But it cannot store what is not in you.

The Larger The Breasts, The More Iodine You Need

Let's say you are a DD cup, the other person is an A, B, or C cup, the larger your breasts the more breasts' tissues you have, so you need a little more iodine because there is more area that requires detoxifying and nourishing. C cup needs more than B and B cup needs more than A cup. But everyone needs it.

Detox Lumps Before They Appear

With proper iodine and selenium, breasts tissue can resist damage, excrete toxins instead of allowing toxins to become lumps. So, you have options: Eat a little seaweed regularly or apply Lugol's to your breasts or ingest Lugol's iodine regularly with selenium. In case you prefer tablets, Ioderol is iodine in tablet form and they are formulated in 12.5 capsules.

Divine Feminine Power

Words are like spells; they can be used manipulatively. For example, what's the difference between mutilation and mastectomy? By cutting, augmenting or irradiating women's breasts, the institutions have violated natural law. Sisters, your breasts are sacred vessels of life, legacy and strength.

You have the power to prevent mastectomy! In case no one has ever told you that during mastectomy procedures, the first step is to cut off the areola, that's the darker area to include the nipples. That part is gone forever. It gets worse - but I am going to stop here. In my opinion this is misogyny – a hatred, a medical way to get away with torturing women legally. Institutions are man made and are not superior to nature or Divine Intelligence.

The Cosmic Recipe was always meant to prevent, restore and maintain our health. Follow the Divine wisdom and recipe that was ORIGINALLY designed and created for you. Then they tell us we are in remission. How can anyone truly be in remission if they never connected with their birthright – the cosmic recipe. When you are in harmony with all of nature at the same time, that's how you maintain your breasts health.

Do you really believe Divine Intelligence devised a system to mutilate you? Many women in the Asian culture eat seaweed, selenium rich foods or supplement selenium to maintain their breast health for life and the same was meant for you too.

Fatigue. Low Energy. Exhausted.

When your body doesn't get enough iodine, your thyroid can't make enough thyroid hormones. That can slow your whole body down and make you feel **very tired**, low-energy, and "dragging" through the day. Getting the **right** amount of iodine (not too little, not too much) helps your thyroid work properly, which can help your energy. (If you have thyroid disease or take meds, talk to a health professional before using iodine.)

Clothing & Skin

- Wear **100% cotton bras and underwear**—natural fabrics breathe, absorb moisture, and reduce risk of infection. Try to avoid underwire if possible.
- Remove your bra at night so your breasts and skin can breathe.
- Choose **aluminum-free deodorants**, since aluminum compounds accumulate in breasts tissues and raise toxic burden.

Vagina & Womb Hygiene

- Use cotton pads or underwear made of natural materials—synthetic fabrics trap heat, moisture and chemicals.
- Avoid powders and sprays in your private area—many contain substances linked to fibroids, uterine issues and cancers.
- During menstruation, don't have sex—let your womb cleanse in peace and avoid introducing all germs, bacteria, toxins or irritants.

Irregular or Heavy Menstrual Cycles

Your ovaries need iodine and potassium iodide to do their job. As egg follicles grow, they use iodine to develop the right way. When a person doesn't get enough iodine, periods can become irregular, and the body may not release an egg every month. That can make it harder to get pregnant. Iodine also supports the ovaries as they make hormones like progesterone, which helps the body prepare for pregnancy.

If your period is heavy or prolonged, your body may be asking for minerals—iodine, potassium iodide, selenium, magnesium or boron.

- **Selenium** neutralizes toxins like mercury *(earth)*
- **Vitamin C** removes fluoride, bromide, and chemical burdens *(earth)*
- **Sea salt** rinses the inner temple *(sea)*
- **Magnesium** helps your body make glutathione—your master cleanser *(sea)*
- **B2 + B3** transport iodine exactly where it needs to go *(earth)*

Together, they form a quiet sisterhood within you. This is Divine breast-care and womb wisdom: **Healing is not a luxury—it is your birthright.**

Story 1: My friend Cassandra experienced a menstrual cycle that lasted nearly a month. During that time, she consistently ate kelp—so much so that it became part of her daily life. One of her favorite snacks was simple and intentional: she would grind together **¼ cup kelp powder, ¼ cup sesame seeds; then and ¼ cup brewer's yeast**, and eat it as is. She shared this snack not only with herself, but with her children as well.

Over time, Cassandra noticed a profound change. The excessive bleeding stopped, and her menstrual cycle gradually returned to what had always been normal for her—three to four days.

This was her lived experience. It was not guided by a prescription, a protocol, or a diagnosis—but by nourishment. Her body responded when it was supplied with what it had been missing.

Note: Eating the kelp snack consistently, Cassandra's children became genius in math and the three have enrolled in engineer, airplane mechanic, and architecture programs in college. The younger children are excelling in advanced math skills too. Read their testimonies in Stolen Intellect 1.

Story 2: Every month Vivi seemed to struggle with her menstrual cycle. One day Vivi's mom called me to say her daughter was on the floor crying what can she do? I said, magnesium worked the last month; did you try that? Mom said, "yes, it didn't work this time." I thought about it, and suggested Camu Camu Vitamin C mixed with MSM.

The next day or so, Vivi called me herself, and was so happy, thankful and appreciative. The mixture worked! Why? Because MSM detoxifies pesticides that accumulate in the body. MSM also relaxes uterine muscle and calms tissue. Vitamin

C lowers inflammation and cramp-triggering prostaglandins —together easing menstrual pain at its source. That day, Vivi became my spiritual daughter!

PMS and Endometriosis

Some doctors, like Dr. Lara Briden, say iodine can help with breast pain, **premenstrual syndrome (PMS)**, **premenstrual dysphoric disorder (PMDD)**, and some ovarian cysts. Iodine helps your body "clean up" estrogen and turns down how loudly estrogen signals in your cells. That's why the right amount of iodine may help with *too-much-estrogen* problems, including endometriosis.

Pain Management

Over time over the counter pain medications can and will compromise your liver. So, try Vitamin C, MSM, and magnesium to manage and minimize your pain. Make them your first option before pain medications. Cramps don't have to be severe and painful. The pain just may be your body letting you know something is missing from your diet.

It's Not The Temperature Outside, But On Your Inside

Thyroid hormones control your body's energy, temperature, and many other jobs. If you don't get enough *iodine*, your thyroid can slow down (hypothyroidism). That can make you feel tired, gain weight, feel cold all the time and have periods that are heavy, light, or irregular.

Why the Struggle to Lose Weight After The Birth

The thyroid relies on iodine to produce its hormones, which regulate metabolism, energy use, and fat burning. When iodine intake is insufficient—especially after pregnancy, when stores have already been depleted—the thyroid can slow down, making postpartum weight loss far more difficult.

Chemicals Surround Us Then Absorb In Us

How do you rinse toxins out your breasts cells and womb before they cause havoc? Iodine – the sea – comes to our rescue and does the internal rinse for us naturally. But depending on where you live, it's not automatic.

Why Eating Lettuce While Pregnant Can Be Dangerous

Greed stripped iodine from our tables while filling our rivers and fields with perchlorate — a rocket-fuel salt that contaminates water, soil, and crops. Dr. David Brownstein warns that lettuce grown in the fall and winter months in the Southwest is often irrigated with perchlorate-contaminated Colorado River water, and that **up to 83% of the nation's fall and winter lettuce supply** comes from that region.

Independent studies confirm that most of America's winter lettuce is produced in the Lower Colorado River basin, where perchlorate has been detected in the river and in lettuce itself. Perchlorate blocks iodine at the thyroid; iodine is the very mineral that helps protect the brain and thyroid from this kind of chemical sabotage.

When people took a dose of the iodine supplement Iodoral (12.5 mg iodide/iodine) for just one day, Dr. Abraham found that in some of them the amount of cadmium in their urine increased many-fold." That means the more cadmium was excreted in the urine, it was no longer in the body.

Bathing on Your Menstrual Cycle

When I was growing up, my mother didn't allow my sisters and me to take tub baths while on our menstrual cycle. She said a woman's body was sacred, and sacred things weren't meant to sit in still water that held what the body had released. That wasn't our way.

Our physical education teachers wouldn't let girls into the swimming pool either. They didn't explain it with big medical terms — they simply taught us that a girl's health was precious, and convenience wasn't worth contamination. The world might say "just get in the water," but our elders taught us to pause, to think, to protect ourselves first.

Tampons

And just because companies made tampons, advertised them, normalized them, and put them in shiny boxes, didn't mean we were free to compromise our principles or our health for a tub or a pool. Our mothers understood things that science is only now catching up to — the microbiome, infection risks, hormonal balance, and the delicate nature of a girl's developing body.

My mother and grandmothers weren't old-fashioned. They were informed — in a way that didn't come from a university, but from generations of women who survived, observed, and passed down their knowledge through care, not commerce.

This is what the Genius Revolution calls **ancestral intelligence**: the wisdom that protected our bodies long before modern systems failed us, the instinct that tells a mother, *"My daughters will not be harmed on my watch,"* the courage to say no to trends that dismiss the sacredness of a girl's biology.

Today, I understand exactly what my mother was doing - She was guarding our future. She was teaching us boundaries. She was preserving the dignity of our developing bodies in a world that markets shortcuts instead of protection.

Our mothers may not have used the word "public health," but they practiced it.

They may not have spoken about hormones, iodine, estrogen balance, or infection prevention, but they lived the truth of them.

Give Your Body The Minerals It Remembers

The more you care for your body, the more faithfully it cares for you. When you nourish it with wisdom and consistency, your days shift from waiting rooms to living rooms—back to the life you were meant to enjoy.

Your options:

- eat seaweed regularly
- ingest Lugol's iodine drops
- apply Lugols iodine directly to the breasts
- use Ioderol tablets
- but, take selenium daily

This is not alternative medicine—it is ancestral medicine.

Dr. Brownstein recommends **25 mg** of iodine daily to detoxify heavy metals. Full Protocol is in his book, *Iodine, Why You Need; Why You Can't Live Without It*.

Note: For my spiritual daughter ViVi, 25 mg is too much. She is small and petite and her body can only handle 6.5 mg. I have larger breasts and have taken 50 mg comfortably for about a month with no problem. Everyone is different. Your size, weight, breasts size matters! Know the protocol before you begin.

It takes a team to maintain thyroid and breasts health

Your team consists of iodine, selenium, iron, zinc, vitamin B12, and vitamin D to do its job. Iodine helps make thyroid hormones, and selenium helps those hormones work safely. Iron and zinc help carry messages through the body, so cells know what to do. Vitamin B12 helps give energy, and vitamin D helps keep the body balanced and healthy. If the body is missing even one of these nutrients, the thyroid may not work well, showing that good thyroid health depends on all six nutrients working together.

The breasts are deeply connected to this process

Breast tissue is highly sensitive to thyroid hormones and iodine, and it relies on a well-functioning thyroid to regulate growth, repair, and maintain hormonal balance. When thyroid hormones are low or disrupted, the breasts may respond with pain, swelling, cysts, tenderness, or abnormal tissue changes. Just like the thyroid, the breasts require iodine for healthy structure, selenium for protection, and vitamin D for proper cell regulation. This is why thyroid imbalance often shows up first in the breasts—and why true breast health begins with nourishing the thyroid.

Note: Sometimes, it can be difficult trying to determine a good iron source and Moringa is a good plant source of iron.

Note: Don't forget Vitamin D rides in on fat. Red palm oil and wheat germ oil **are** two of the most powerful nutrient-delivery oils on earth when used correctly.

Remember: Don't Just Check Your Breasts for Lumps – Prevent the Lumps

Starting in our teenage years, healthcare institutions guided us girls to regularly examine our breasts for any lumps. But Matriarchy — the original teacher — would have asked a different question: *How do we prevent the lumps from forming in the first place?*

Basic breast care is not merely early detection.

It is **prevention**, nourishment, and wisdom passed through the Divine Feminine from generation to generation:

Iodine for the breasts tissue.

Selenium for protection.

Vitamin A and E for healing.

Other sea minerals for balance.

This is the heart of **B.B.I.B.L.E** — *Basic Breastcare Instructions Before Leaving Earth*:

Not fear, but foresight.

Not panic, but prevention.

Not waiting for disease, but building health long before disease has the opportunity to exist.

Before clocks and empires, time was kept in 28 days—the moon, the womb, and the waters moving as one.

CHAPTER 30 BIBLIOGRAPHY

1. **Mathews, D. M.** "Iodine and Fertility: Do We Know Enough?" *Human Reproduction* (2021). Oxford University Press.
2. **Mills, J. L., et al.** "Delayed Conception in Women with Low Urinary Iodine Concentrations." *Human Reproduction* 33, no. 3 (2018): 481–489. Oxford University Press.
3. **National Institutes of Health, Office of Dietary Supplements.** "Iodine — Consumer Fact Sheet." NIH Office of Dietary Supplements. https://ods.od.nih.gov.
4. **U.S. Department of Health and Human Services, Office on Women's Health.** "Thyroid Disease." Office on Women's Health. https://womenshealth.gov.
5. **Briden, Lara.** "Why I Prescribe Iodine for Breast Pain, Ovarian Cysts, and Premenstrual Mood Symptoms." *The Period Revolutionary* (2025). https://larabriden.com.
6. **Maine Coast Sea Vegetables.** "Dulse Seaweed Nutrition Profile." Maine Coast Sea Vegetables.
7. **Axe, Josh (Dr. Axe).** "Dulse: Nutrition, Benefits, and Uses." DrAxe.com.
8. **Dr. David Brownstein.** *"Iodine: Why You Need It, Why You Can't Live Without It"* (West Bloomfield, MI: Medical Alternatives Press, 2009).
9. **Shulhai, Andreea M., et al.** "The Role of Nutrition on Thyroid Function." *Nutrients* 16, no. 15 (2024): 2496. https://doi.org/10.3390/nu16152496.
10. **Duntas, Leonidas H.** "Nutrition and Thyroid Disease." *Journal of Thyroid Research* (2023): Article ID 8753493. https://doi.org/10.1155/2023/8753493.

CHAPTER 31

THE PROSTATE PROTECTION CODE

When you nourish the man, you restore the lineage;
when you restore the lineage, you heal the nation.

Brothers, never stop fighting for your health. Even when the diagnosis feels heavy, never hand over your hope. No institution and no expert can write the ending to your story. Not now. Not ever.

If you feel like you've tried everything, it simply means it's time to try something different. Keep going. Your body wants to heal—and it will meet you halfway.

Erectile Dysfunction Resolved at 60 Years Old

Mr. RJ and I first connected on TikTok in 2025. He in-boxed me. "I'm 60," he said. "Do you think you can help me with erectile dysfunction?"

"Absolutely," I told him. "It should not take long for the supplements to work. Once they are in your system, I envision you waking up to a full erection."

About a week after starting the protocol, my phone rang.

"Guess what?" he said, laughing like a surprised teenager. "The supplements worked! I hope it's not too much information to tell you I woke up hard."

I celebrated with him, because one thing about RJ—he **listened**, and he followed every instruction with discipline.

Here's a list of the supplements he took:

- **Red Palm Oil** – rich in natural Vitamin E and Vitamin A to strengthen circulation and immunity.
- **Organic Camu Camu Vitamin C + MSM** – to help detoxify pesticide residue ("roach spray") from fruits and vegetables. A teaspoon a day cleanses what the body cannot remove alone.

- **Selenium (link in the rear)** – he took two capsules daily and continues to do so.
- **B1/B6/B12 tincture** – to support nerve function and energy.
- **J. Crows Lugol's Iodine 2%** – 5 small drops in ¼ cup of water every day (12 mg) to restore thyroid and hormonal balance.
- **Magnesium (2 tablets at night)** – essential for rest and repair. As a truck driver, deep sleep helped his body heal.

He changed his toothpaste, too—because everything is relative.

RJ also made intentional lifestyle shifts. He began preparing meals at home, choosing avocados and fresh fruits, and avoiding fast food as much as possible—even while traveling. These choices supported his hormones, improved circulation, and strengthened his body's capacity to recover.

Within days, his body responded. RJ healed himself by feeding what had been starved—allowing his cells to remember their original instructions.

Ozone Water and Prostate Health

Another overlooked remedy for circulation and prostate health is ozone-infused water. Ozone oxygenates water, kills bacteria and viruses, increases oxygen flow through the body, lowers blood pressure, and improves circulation. A simple ozone machine, called A2Z, can cost less than $90.

One of my friends—who had long struggled with impotence—shared that he felt noticeable improvements after drinking ozonated water daily for several weeks. He described the water as fresh and energizing and said it helped him feel more revitalized and better oxygenated overall. In his words, it brought life back into his body and restored a sense of strength, confidence, and manhood he hadn't felt in years.

Beets for Blood Flow and Erection

High blood pressure and erectile dysfunction (ED) are medically linked. Beets are nature's blood-pressure medicine. They contain dietary nitrates which the body converts into nitric oxide—a gas that dilates blood vessels, improves circulation, and relaxes the smooth muscle tissue required for erection. More blood flow = more life force. Something as simple as beet-juice or beet supplements can restore vitality to the body.

Why Men Should Especially Eat Barnyard Millet

Barnyard Millet:

- Improves blood flow by lowering cholesterol
- Stabilizes blood sugar so testosterone rises
- Reduces inflammation that constricts arteries
- Helps the body burn fat instead of storing it
- Supports the heart — the engine of circulation
- For a man, improved circulation = improved erections, vitality, strength, and mood.

Note: *Always buy dehulled, unpolished millet* as the gold standard.
Unpolished = whole nutrition.
Dehulled = digestible.
Together = the most powerful form.

New Car Interiors — A Silent Assault on Your Prostate

That "new car smell" so many people love is actually a chemical warning. The scent comes from volatile compounds — including **brominated chemicals similar to potassium bromate**, plasticizers, and flame retardants — all off-gassing into the air you breathe.

Now imagine this:
You **eat toxic bromate** in bread…
You **inhale brominated fumes** during your commute…

That "luxury scent" you inhale is not perfume — it is a chemical warning. Those same volatile compounds settle into your bloodstream, your lungs, your lymph, your reproductive organs.

They don't just fade; they accumulate. And for a man already battling inflammation, hormonal imbalance, or prostate distress, this becomes silent sabotage.

Consider the pathway:

- You inhale toxic compounds in the morning commute.
- You consume potassium-bromate-treated bread at lunch.
- You sit in a heated car seat releasing more chemicals on the way home.

- Or you drive a brand new RV wreaking with potassium bromate during the day then sleep in the toxic fumes at night.

One day becomes years. Years become a lifetime. And the prostate — a small gland with a massive role — is forced to absorb blow after blow.

This is why prostate conditions seem to "appear out of nowhere." They don't. They are built, layer by layer, through constant exposure to toxins no one warned you about.

But here is the good news:

The body remembers how to repair itself when you return to the elements that formed it — Lugol's iodine, selenium, magnesium, Vitamin E, antioxidants, whole foods, sea minerals, rest, and sunlight.

The prostate is not doomed.

It is waiting for restoration.

And when you remove the silent attackers — the toxic bread, the toxic air, the toxic environment — you give your body permission to heal.

You reclaim your strength.

Your clarity.

Your vitality.

Your drive.

Because a toxic world may shape a man's struggle…

but a nourished body rewrites his destiny.

In Closing

I wrote this chapter with one intention: to return power to your hands. Health was never meant to be a maze — it was meant to be elemental, rooted in earth, air, sea, and sun. I do not believe in disease; I believe in the power of the firmament and in the body's ability to heal when it is given what it has always needed.

A man's prostate was designed to remain strong, resilient, and vibrant at every age. When we restore the elements, restoration follows. When we return to what remembers us, the body answers.

May this chapter guide you back to strength, clarity, and wholeness — because your health was never meant to decline; it was meant to rise.

CHAPTER 31 BIBLIOGRAPHY

1. Beetroot & Nitric Oxide. *The Potential Benefits of Red Beetroot Supplementation in Health and Disease.* PubMed Central (PMC).
2. Healthline. "Beet Juice and Erectile Dysfunction: Can Nitrates Help?" *Healthline.com.*
3. Ugare, R., Chimmad, B., Rajyalakshmi, P., et al. "Nutritional and Functional Significance of Barnyard Millet (*Echinochloa frumentacea*): A Review." *Karnataka Journal of Agricultural Sciences* 24, no. 4 (2011): 583–585.
4. Ugare, R., Chimmad, B., Naik, R., Bharati, P., & Itagi, S. "Glycemic Index and Significance of Barnyard Millet (*Echinochloa frumentacea*) in Type 2 Diabetes." *Journal of Food Science and Technology* (2011).
5. Kumari, P., and B. Thayumanavan. "Studies on Barnyard Millet Starch for Dietary Management of Diabetics." *Journal of Food Science and Technology* 34, no. 4 (1997): 281–283.

CHAPTER 32

PENIS PAINTING

Over the years, I have come across many natural remedies—some passed down through families, others quietly shared in small corners of the health community. A few may seem unusual at first, but once you understand the stories and the science behind them, their wisdom becomes clear.

One such remedy was described by two young men who noticed meaningful improvements in their strength and vitality after using a simple topical mixture. Their testimony could have easily been overlooked, but I felt it deserved to be shared—for the many men who silently struggle and may benefit from knowing that gentle, natural options exist.

The Penis Painting Recipe

You only need two ingredients:

1. J. Crow's Lugol's 2% iodine
2. Grapeseed oil

How to Prepare:

- Mix about 1 teaspoon of grapeseed oil into ¾ bottle of J. Crow's Lugol's iodine.
- Shake well.
- Be careful: iodine can stain towels, floors, ceramic, and clothing. Apply it carefully.

Application Instructions

- **Day 1**: Apply the mixture across the **top** of the penis, from the pubic hairline to the tip (but not inside the urethra, as this may cause burning). Let it dry completely.
- **Day 2**: Apply the mixture to the **underside** of the penis, from the anus to the tip (again avoiding the urethra).
- **Day 3**: Alternate back to the top and continue rotating daily.

This alternating application supports detoxification, helps excrete toxic buildup, and may restore circulation and strength to a man's reproductive system.

Penis Painting Testimonies

I prepared bottles of this recipe and mailed them out to several male friends—only to those in relationships—because I knew if it worked, their partners would notice too.

- **Brother in his 60s**: One of my friends, in his early 60s, tried the mixture. He told me it worked for him, but even more convincing was his girlfriend's reaction: she noticed his erection lasted longer than before. To his surprise, while using the product, his wife became pregnant. He was already taking sea moss, but he was convinced that penis painting was the real key.
- **Another friend**: This brother didn't give me details about his partner but said enthusiastically that the product worked for him and improved his strength and vitality.
- **Online testimonies**: The original two young men who shared this recipe on Curezone both reported stronger erections and improved stamina after consistent use.

A Word of Wisdom

I am here to urge you—do not give up on yourself.

Do not abandon the fight for your health, your strength, or your future. This is not medical advice; it is a quiet invitation to every brother to nourish his body the way nature intended.

Remember this truth: every man is born through the womb of a woman. If her thyroid was weary, if her iodine and selenium were stolen or scarce, then her son entered the world with the same missing elements. But restoration is your birthright.

When a man begins to return what has been taken—**iodine, selenium, red palm oil, and the minerals of the ocean**—his body remembers its original design. His strength rises. His clarity sharpens. His courage returns.

In giving your body back its elements, you reclaim not only your health, but your vitality, your manhood, and the legacy waiting behind your name.

CHAPTER 32 BIBLIOGRAPHY

1. Carani, C., et al. "Multicenter Study on the Prevalence of Sexual Symptoms in Male Hypo- and Hyperthyroid Patients." *Journal of Clinical Endocrinology & Metabolism* 90, no. 12 (2005): 6472–6479.
   Findings: Sexual dysfunction, including erectile dysfunction, is common in both hypothyroid and hyperthyroid patients and often improves after restoration of euthyroid status.

CHAPTER 33

A NOTE TO BOY MOMS

Our families are under attack. Our sons—the boys we cradle, raise, and prepare for manhood—are growing up in a world where preventable health crises quietly rob men of their vitality. One of the most devastating is prostate disease.

By 2025, projections showed that more than **350 million male teens and men worldwide** would suffer prostate problems—more than the entire population of the United States. Prior to 2025, prostate problems were at 30 million statistically. The scale feels unthinkable, yet much of this suffering is preventable.

And here is the truth many mothers never hear:

A mother holds the power to nourish and protect her son's prostate long before disease ever begins.

Nourish the Boy, Protect the Man

A mother begins shaping her son's health from the moment his heartbeat sparks beneath hers. Every mineral she absorbs, every nutrient she restores, every sea-born gift she returns to her body becomes the quiet foundation of her son's future strength.

Women are told they shape daughters—wombs, cycles, hormones. But few are told this: **Mothers shape their sons too.**

They shape his prostate.

They shape his hormonal balance.

They shape his future fertility and manhood.

Infertility does not begin at midlife—it begins in childhood, in the years when missing minerals quietly weaken the body from the inside out.

But mothers are not powerless.

They are the first healers their children will ever know.

With every mineral they restore, they secure a legacy.

A mother's nourishment is more than food.

It is inheritance.

The Diabetes–Prostate Connection

Emerging research reveals something profound:
Vitamin D deficiency and low ocean minerals in childhood raise the risk of Type 1 diabetes, which can later contribute to erectile dysfunction and reproductive decline in adulthood.

A major review showed children with Type 1 diabetes had **up to 50% lower Vitamin D levels** than healthy children. Older research suggested that cod liver oil in infancy reduced Type 1 diabetes risk, though guidelines have since shifted.

Today, the safest approach is:

- **Babies under 12 months:** vitamin D drops only
- **Children 1 year and older:** small daily doses of cod liver oil if needed
- **Check vitamin A and D levels to avoid excess**
- **Always follow age-appropriate dosing**

Cod liver oil remains a powerful source of nutrients children lack today:

- *Omega-3s for the brain and heart*
- *Vitamin D for immunity and hormone balance*
- *Vitamin A for vision and growth*

Prevention Through Nourishment (The Mother's Shield)

Boy moms can create lifelong protection by weaving these essentials into daily life:

Cod Liver Oil (after age 1)

Supports intelligence, vision, hormones, immunity.

Iodine & Seaweed

Wakame, kelp, bladderwrack—boost metabolism, protect reproductive organs, support thyroid and prostate health.

Selenium (preferably SelenoExcell)

A cancer shield; essential for prostate health and hormone balance.

Red Palm Oil

Full-spectrum Vitamin A and E for brain, eyes, skin, and immunity.
These are not trends—they are tools.
Mothers who nourish their sons early are building:

- stronger prostates
- healthier hormones
- sharper cognition
- protected fertility
- resilience against diabetes and ED

A mother's nourishment today prevents a man's suffering decades from now.

A Broken System

Other nations run prevention programs: monitoring iodine, fortifying foods, teaching families how to protect their children.
But in the U.S., prevention is not a priority.
Appointments exist, but prevention programs do not.
And so deficiencies grow into epidemics, leaving millions of men vulnerable.

What the Body Was Trying to Communicate

A classmate of mine passed recently from Type 1 diabetes and cancer. Before he transitioned, he left a peaceful message online—a goodbye full of gratitude. But reading it through the lens of mineral wisdom, what I heard was this:

The original message said: I am dying of Type 1 Diabetes and Caner. I am surrounded by my family. I had a beautiful life and I am in hospice and wanted to say goodbye to my classmates before I go.....

I cried many times after reading my classmates Facebook post because what I heard was this:
"I lived a beautiful life...
but my body did not receive enough sun and ended up with Type 1 Diabetes.

I did not receive the ocean minerals designed to protect and regenerate me, and I became overwhelmed with toxins that caused cancer.

And now I must go."

His passing awakened something in me—not fear, but clarity. As a boy mom, you carry the quiet power to shape your son's future strength, to guard his manhood before he even understands the word "man."

With minerals from the ocean, vitamins from the soil, oils from the palm, and iodine from the sea, you are building a shield around him that lasts long after childhood fades.

May your love nourish his cells, may your wisdom protect his prostate, and may your care echo forward into the men and fathers your sons are destined to become. Our boys need protection long before adulthood. And mothers hold that power.

Mothers, You Are Your Son's First Line of Defense

Long before the world names him, tests him, educates him, or challenges him—**you nourish him.**

The Most High chose you to carry him, strengthen him, and shield him. This is why:

A mother is the first prevention program her son will ever have. Prevention is her superpower.

Your son's future begins with you.

And you are more powerful than you know.

CHAPTER 33 BIBLIOGRAPHY

1. Hay, G. (2020). "New Advice on Vitamin D Supplements and Cod Liver Oil for Infants." *Tidsskriftet for Den norske legeforening* (The Journal of the Norwegian Medical Association).
   Note: Reports updated national guidance stating that cod liver oil is no longer recommended during the first year of life; breastfed infants should still receive vitamin D supplementation.
2. Helsenorge. "Vitamin Supplements (Infants)." Norway's official public health portal.

3. Norwegian Directorate of Health (Helsedirektoratet). *Food and Meals for Infants* (English PDF).
4. Cortese, M. M., et al. (2015). "Timing of Use of Cod Liver Oil, a Vitamin D Source, and Risk of Disease."

If prevention is love in action, what do we call it when there is no prevention?

A setup.
A sabotage.
A system designed to watch us break.

CHAPTER 34

MOTHER NATURE'S PHARMACY

The *ocean* and the *earth* have always been our greatest pharmacies. From the depths of the sea to the roots of the forest, nature placed healing compounds in plants, minerals, and fungi to nourish, protect, and restore us. Two of the most profound natural healers we can add to our diet are **seaweed** and the **Agaricus Blazei mushroom**.

Seaweed: Ocean Intelligence for the Body

Seaweed is not just food—it is medicine hidden in plain sight. There are three main types:

- **Red Seaweed** – Rich in protein, antioxidants, and phytonutrients.
- **Brown Seaweed** – The most widely consumed, including Mozuku, Wakame (Mekabu), and Kombu (kelp). This variety contains the powerful compound fucoidan.
- **Green Seaweed** – Abundant in chlorophyll and minerals that detoxify and energize the body.

What is Fucoidan?

Research shows it has profound effects on cell health, immune function, and tumor suppression. It works on a cellular level, supporting **apoptosis** (suicide for damaged cells) while protecting and nourishing healthy ones.

Research tip: If you want to dig into studies on fucoidan's role in cancer prevention, search for **"fucoidan"** rather than "cancer." A wealth of data opens up—much of it overlooked in conventional medical treatment.

Documented Benefits of Fucoidan

Studies have highlighted fucoidan's ability to suppress tumor growth and strengthen the body's natural defense system, showing anti-tumor potential against:

- Colon tumors
- Breast tumors
- Lung tumors
- Liver cancer (hepatoma)
- Leukemia
- Bladder tumors
- Multiple other cancer types

Beyond fucoidan, seaweed is naturally high in **iodine** and is both a **nutritional powerhouse** and a **protective shield.**

The Power of Seaweed

In East Asia—especially Japan and Korea—seaweed dishes made from wakame, hijiki, and kombu are staple foods. These ocean vegetables embody Hippocrates' wisdom: *"Let food be thy medicine."* They prevent disease, strengthen health, and increase longevity.

The more seaweed we eat, the lower rates of diabetes, heart disease, obesity, high cholesterol, high blood pressure, stroke, and gut problems. Seaweed is also a natural immune supporter.

HIV and Immune System

In fact, research shows that **wakame and spirulina can strengthen immune systems in people living with HIV** by boosting white blood cell activity and reducing oxidative stress (Selmi et al., 2011; Ramamoorthy & Premakumari, 1996).

This means that the same foods that extend life in healthy populations can bring resilience and strength to those facing serious immune challenges.

Adding wakame and kombu to our diet is not just a health upgrade—it is an answered prayer for disease prevention and longevity.

Immune Resilience — Seaweed + Spirulina for HIV Support

For people living with HIV, the immune system is under constant strain. But research shows that nature provides allies in unexpected places.

- **Wakame (brown seaweed)** delivers **fucoidan**, a compound that strengthens immune defense and reduces inflammation.
- **Spirulina (blue-green algae)** contains proteins and antioxidants that **stimulate white blood cells, boost natural killer cell activity, and reduce oxidative stress.**

Clinical trials have found that spirulina can improve immune function in HIV-positive individuals, increasing resilience and quality of life (Selmi et al., 2011; Ramamoorthy & Premakumari, 1996). When combined with wakame, this duo becomes more than nutrition—it is **a daily act of immune empowerment.**

Seaweed delivers the ocean's iodine and trace minerals. Spirulina, though freshwater-grown, supplies iron, protein, and protective pigments. Together they form a complementary water-grown pairing.

Message of Hope: Seaweed and spirulina are not exotic luxuries; they are accessible, life-giving foods that can change the story of health.

Healing Seaweeds

Wakame (Brown Seaweed)

- Antioxidant – fights harmful free radicals linked to chronic disease.
- Anti-inflammatory – reduces harmful inflammation.
- Anti-cancer – helps arrest or prevent tumor growth.
- Anti-hypertensive (helps lower blood pressure) and supports healthy blood pressure (critical since ~50% of U.S. adults live with hypertension).
- Antidiabetic – balances blood sugar and helps prevent complications.
- Antiviral – protects against infections.
- Anticoagulant – reduces risk of clots, stroke, and heart attack.
- Anti-osteoporotic – supports bone strength.
- Hepatoprotective – protects the liver.
- Anti-obesity – helps manage weight and fat metabolism.

Kombu (Brown Seaweed)

- Anticoagulant & Antithrombotic – protects the heart and circulation.
- Anti-cancer – supports defense against abnormal cell growth.
- Hypolipidemic – lowers cholesterol.
- Hypoglycemic – regulates blood sugar and supports diabetes prevention.
- Anti-obesity – reduces risk of weight-related illness.
- Anti-atherosclerosis – slows plaque buildup in arteries.
- Renal protective – supports kidney health.
- Vascular protective – guards against blood vessel damage.
- Antioxidant – protects against oxidative stress.
- Antimicrobial – fights harmful bacteria, viruses, and fungi.
- Anti-inflammatory – calms chronic inflammation.
- Immunomodulatory – strengthens immune balance.
- Gut biota regulatory – supports a healthy gut microbiome.
- Neuroprotective – protects and preserves brain cells.

Suppress Tumor Developoment/Support Immune strength

This is worth pointing out. Let us return to **fucoidan**, a sulfated polysaccharide found primarily in brown seaweed. Fucoidan has been widely studied for its ability to **support immune strength and regulate abnormal cell growth**, including mechanisms that suppress tumor development.

Its power lies not in force, but in design—sulfated sugar chains that communicate with the body, guiding immune cells, calming inflammation, and restoring order where chaos threatens life.

This is not accidental chemistry. It is **Divine Intelligence encoded in the sea**, offering protection, balance, and defense to those who remember how to receive it.

What These Two Words Really Mean - "Sulfated" and "Polysaccharide"

Sulfated are sulfate groups—made from *sulfur and oxygen*—are attached to those sugar chains. This sulfation gives the molecule a negative electrical charge, allowing it to bind water, interact with cells, regulate inflammation and communicate biologically. Without sulfation, many polysaccharides are inactive; with sulfation, they become *protective and functional.*

Sulfation makes molecules:

- More **water-soluble**
- More **biologically active**
- Better able to **communicate with cells**
- Protective rather than irritating

*Sulfation is not decoration—it is **activation**.*

A **polysaccharide** is a long chain of natural sugars linked together. Unlike simple sugars that spike blood sugar, polysaccharides act as **structural and communication molecules** in the body. They form gels, scaffolding, and protective barriers that support the brain, gut, joints, blood vessels, and immune system.

In short: **polysaccharides build the structure—sulfation turns them on.**

Sulfated Polysaccharides: What They Are

Polysaccharides are long chains of sugars that form the **structural and communication matrix of life**—think of them as biological scaffolding and messaging cables.

When polysaccharides are **sulfated**, they become some of the most powerful biological compounds known.

Common **sulfated polysaccharides** include:

- **Fucoidan** (brown seaweed)
- **Carrageenan** (red seaweed)
- **Agar**
- **Heparan sulfate**
- **Chondroitin sulfate**
- **Keratan sulfate**

These are not supplements invented in a lab—they are **foundational molecules of human tissue.**

Why Sulfation Matters in the Body

Sulfated polysaccharides:

- Carry **negative electrical charges**
- Bind water like a gel
- Create **cushioning, lubrication, and protection**

- Regulate **cell signaling, immunity, and inflammation**

This is why they are abundant in:

- **Brain tissue**
- **Cartilage and joints**
- **Blood vessels**
- **Skin**
- **The gut lining**

Without sulfation, tissues dry out, stiffen, inflame, and lose resilience.

Sulfated Polysaccharides & the Brain

In the brain, sulfated polysaccharides:

- Help form the **extracellular matrix**
- Guide **neuronal growth and wiring**
- Regulate **synaptic communication**
- Protect neurons from toxins and inflammation

This is why iodine, sulfur, selenium, and ocean minerals matter—they support the **sulfation pathways** that keep the brain flexible and protected.

A brain without proper sulfation is like wiring without insulation.

The Ocean Connection

Seaweeds are rich in **pre-sulfated polysaccharides**, meaning:

- The body doesn't have to struggle to make them
- They arrive **already activated**
- They restore tissues gently and efficiently

This is why traditional coastal cultures:

- Had stronger joints
- Better immunity
- Healthier pregnancies

- Sharper cognition

They were literally **eating the extracellular matrix of the sea.**

What Happens When Sulfation Is Low

When sulfation pathways are impaired:

- Detoxification slows
- Inflammation rises
- Cartilage degenerates
- Blood vessels stiffen
- Brain signaling weakens

Modern diets low in sulfur, iodine, and marine foods **starve the body of sulfation.**

This is not aging.

This is **biochemical neglect.**

Agaricus Blazei Mushroom: Earth's Immune Guardian

Known as the **"Mushroom of the Gods"** in its native Brazil. Agaricus Blazei has earned worldwide respect for its immune-boosting and medicinal properties. Paired with seaweed, it creates a synergy that strengthens both mind and body.

Seaweed + Mushrooms

When seaweed's **fucoidan compounds** join forces with Agaricus Blazei's **immune-boosting polysaccharides**, the result is a natural alliance against inflammation, viral threats, and abnormal cell growth. This ocean-and-earth partnership provides nourishment, detoxification, and long-term protection *that no synthetic drug can match.*

It is not a typical culinary mushroom — it is prized for its *medicinal compounds.*

Blazei Mushroom

1. Immune System Strengthening

Agaricus Blazei is rich in **β-glucans**, compounds that activate and strengthen immune cells such as:

- macrophages
- natural killer (NK) cells
- T-cells

Your Body's Immune Team.
Your immune system is like a **security team** that protects your body every day.

Macrophages

Macrophages are the **clean-up crew**. They find germs, bacteria, and damaged cells and **eat them**. After cleaning up, they warn the rest of the immune system that trouble is nearby.

Natural Killer (NK) Cells

NK cells are the **first responders**. They look for cells that don't belong—like virus-infected or cancer cells—and **destroy them quickly** before they cause more harm.

T-Cells

T-cells are the **commanders and soldiers**. Some T-cells tell the immune system when to attack, some fight germs directly, and others remember past infections so your body can respond faster next time.

2. Anti-Cancer Support (Adjunct, not a Cure)

Studies suggest ABM may help:

- reduce tumor growth
- enhance the effectiveness of chemotherapy
- protect healthy cells from damage

3. Anti-Inflammatory Properties

Agaricus Blazei helps lower systemic inflammation, which benefits people with:

- autoimmune issues
- chronic inflammation
- metabolic disease

- cardiovascular disease

4. Blood Sugar Regulation

This makes it interesting for people with *prediabetes, diabetes, or metabolic syndrome.*

5. Liver Protection

ABM has hepatoprotective effects — helping the liver detoxify toxins and protect it from damage caused by:

- alcohol
- medications
- oxidative stress

6. Antiviral and Antimicrobial Effects

The mushroom contains compounds that inhibit certain viruses and bacteria, supporting the body's natural defense systems.

Who Might Benefit Most

ABM is often used by:

- individuals seeking immune strength
- cancer patients (as a complementary therapy)
- people with chronic inflammation
- diabetics or pre-diabetics
- those needing liver support
- people prone to infections

Note: Agaricus Blazei is available as whole dried mushrooms, powdered form, capsules, hot-water extracts, and tinctures. For immune benefits, extracts or dual-extracted tinctures deliver the most concentrated beta-glucans, while whole mushrooms offer the full natural profile.

My Personal Seaweed Testimonies

While researching seaweed, I came across a fascinating study: when rice was eaten alone, blood sugar levels spiked. But when rice was eaten with seaweed—or when seaweed was eaten first—the blood-sugar rise was significantly blunted. It struck me then: perhaps we have been eating rice, carbohydrates, and starches the wrong way all along.

Yes, these foods should be eaten in moderation. But when they are enjoyed, pairing them with seaweed appears to support metabolic balance. The order of our food matters.

One day, I had the opportunity to test this insight for myself. After eating a piece of watermelon, I felt a sharp pain shoot through my toe. It wasn't rice—but the natural sugars in the watermelon produced a similar reaction. In that moment, the study came rushing back to me.

I walked to my refrigerator and took out a bowl of wakame salad I had prepared earlier. I reached for a small piece of wakame seaweed, chewed it slowly, and swallowed. Within seconds, the pain in my foot eased. My blood sugar had settled that quickly. Nori seaweed with rice should be just as effective and enjoyable too.

Sisters, this is my point: we must change how we eat. It is not enough to talk about health—we must practice it, beginning in our own kitchens. Small portions of seaweed added to home-cooked meals can make a meaningful difference over time.

Recently, my daughter sent me a photo of her dinner: a steaming bowl of red lentil soup with just a small amount of wakame placed in the center. I smiled. She is learning—and she is teaching my grandchildren how to prepare and enjoy wakame seaweed as well.

My grandson, only twelve years old, genuinely loves wakame salad. I cannot help but notice how well he is performing in his math class. One day, he told me that two teachers had remarked on his intelligence. When I asked which teachers, he replied, "My math teachers." I smiled again.

This is not coincidence.

This is nourishment.

This is how we restore brilliance and health—one meal at a time.

Reflection: The Creator's Pharmacy

These are not accidents; they are provisions. They whisper to us even now: *healing is possible, balance can be restored, and strength can return to our generations.*

CHAPTER 34 BIBLIOGRAPHY

1. **Selmi, C., et al.** "Spirulina and Immune Function: A Randomized Clinical Trial in Healthy Volunteers and HIV Patients." *Journal of Medicinal Food* 14, no. 9 (2011): 1130–1137.

2. **Ramamoorthy, A., and S. Premakumari.** "Effect of Spirulina on the Immune Status of HIV-Infected Individuals." *Journal of Nutritional Science and Vitaminology* 42, no. 4 (1996): 373–381.

3. **Fitton, J. H.** "Therapies from Fucoidan: Multifunctional Marine Polymers." *Marine Drugs* 9, no. 10 (2011): 1731–1760.

4. **Hetland, G., et al.** "The Mushroom *Agaricus Blazei Murill*: Immunomodulatory Effects and Clinical Studies." *Phytotherapy Research* 25, no. 8 (2011): 1115–1121.

5. **Mouritsen, O. G., et al.** "Seaweed for Umami and Nutrition in the New Nordic Cuisine." *Flavour* 2, no. 17 (2013).

6. **Keegan, R. J., et al.** "Vitamin D2 from UV-Irradiated Mushrooms Is Safe, Bioavailable, and Effectively Raises Serum 25(OH)D Concentrations." *Journal of Nutrition* 143, no. 5 (2013): 541–547.

EPILOGUE

THE GENIUS REVOLUTION & HEALING MOVEMENT BEGINS

Before nations had borders, before governments had ministries, before science had language,
   there was the sea.
   The first cradle of minerals.
   The first whisper of intelligence.
   The first pulse of the elements that shaped our bodies, our minds, our memory, our destiny.
   Long before we called it "iodine,"
   it was the quiet architect of brilliance
   woven into the oceans,
   woven into our mothers,
   woven into the very blueprint of life.
   And somewhere along the journey—
   between empire and industry,
   between migration and survival,
   between policy and neglect—
   we forgot.
   Not because we were careless,
   but because we were overwhelmed.
   Generations pushed into survival mode
   do not always have the luxury of remembering
   the science that once belonged to our grandmothers' kitchens and our ancestors' oceanlands.
   Yet memory has a rhythm.
   Wisdom has a tide.

Truth has a way of rising again.
And now, in your hands, a revolution rises!
Not the kind forged in noise and conflict—
but in clarity.
In nourishment.
In restoration.
In the unshakable belief that intelligence is our birthright
and wellness is our inheritance.
This book is not an ending;
it is our rebirth, our genesis.
A return to Divine Intelligence—
the cosmic instructions written into every cell.
A return to stewardship—
the sacred responsibility to protect what we carry.
A return to the table—
where mothers reclaim their strength,
fathers reclaim their guidance,
children reclaim their genius,
and families reclaim their future.
For far too long, deficiency disguised itself as destiny.
Symptoms masqueraded as disease.
And deficiency was misdiagnosed as failure.
But here you stand—
a witness, a messenger, a guardian—
ready to break that cycle.
Because once you know what the elements do,
you cannot unknow it.
Once you taste restoration,
you cannot pretend you are powerless.
Once you see the generations waking up,
you cannot return to sleep.
You have seen with your own eyes
that a teaspoon of iodized salt
can change a lifetime.
A drop of cod liver oil
can reshape a lineage.
A mineral restored

can restore an entire nation.
This is the quiet revolution within the human story—
that healing does not always require a hospital,
change does not always require permission,
and intelligence does not always come from institutions.
Sometimes, it comes from the ocean.
Sometimes, it comes from the land.
Sometimes, it comes from a mother who refuses to quit.
And sometimes—
it comes through you.
You are entering a movement older than textbooks
and wiser than politics—
a movement made of people who choose clarity over confusion,
courage over fear,
and generational health over generational harm.
This is the Genius Revolution.
A rising of minds,
a repairing of wombs,
a remembering of truth,
a rebirth of nations—
one family at a time.
And as you close this chapter,
know this:
You carry the future every time you nourish your body.
You protect a lineage every time you choose iodized salt.
You strengthen a nation every time you teach someone what you now know.
You change destiny every time you feed a child from the ocean's wisdom.
The world may not understand the magnitude of this moment,
but generations from now,
your descendants will.
They will inherit sharper minds,
healthier bodies,
steadier spirits,
and dreams their grandparents never had permission to imagine.
They will know that **you**
—yes, you—
were the hinge of history.

THE GENIUS REVOLUTION & HEALING MOVEMENT BEGINS

The bridge between what was lost
and what is now restored.
The living proof that when a single parent,
a single teacher,
a single leader,
a single soul wakes up—
entire nations begin to rise.
So let this be your final reminder:
You are Minerallymade.
Not disease-made.
Not deficiency-made.
Not fear-made.

You are the continuation of Divine Cosmic Intelligence, experiencing life in human form, carrying the power to repair and protect every fractured generation yet to come. The Cosmic Recipe is for us all to remember.

And the revolution?
It begins now.
It begins with you.
It begins at your table.
And the world will never be the same.

~ **The Beginning** ~

The true meaning of a matriarchal civilization

*The power of Matriarchy was never meant
to compete with masculinity.
It is the quiet architecture of life—women holding the
rhythms of birth, nourishment, and continuity, while
men guard, build, and extend what is born.
Together, they form the design.*

SELECTED REFERENCES & FURTHER READING

Iodine & Brain Development

- Velasco, Bath & Rayman (2018). *Iodine as an essential nutrient during the first 1000 days of life.* Nutrients.
- Lee et al. (2017). *Iodine contents in prenatal vitamins in the United States.* Thyroid.
- Zimmermann (2009). *Iodine deficiency in pregnancy and the effects of maternal iodine supplementation on the offspring.* American Journal of Clinical Nutrition.

Choline & Pregnancy

- NIH Office of Dietary Supplements (2025). *Dietary Supplements and Life Stages: Pregnancy.*
- Korsmo et al. (2019). *Choline: Exploring the growing science on its benefits for moms & babies.* Nutrients.

Selenium, Vitamin E & Thyroid Function

- Kohrle (2025). *Thyroid hormones, selenium, and functional hypothyroidism: A review.* Biological Trace Element Research.
- Salonen et al. (1998). *Effect of Vitamin E and Selenium on Atherosclerosis in Mice.* Circulation Research.
- Rayman (2012). *Selenium and human health.* The Lancet.

Environmental Toxins & Maternal Health

- Gardener et al. (2025). *Heavy metals and phthalate contamination in prenatal vitamins.* American Journal of Clinical Nutrition.
- Lisco et al. (2020). *Interference on iodine uptake and human thyroid function by environmental pollutants.* International Journal of Molecular Sciences.

- ACOG Committee Opinion No. 803 (2021). *Reducing Prenatal Exposure to Toxic Environmental Agents.* Obstetrics & Gynecology.
- CDC (2024). *Lead and Breastfeeding.*

Nutrition & Global Literacy

- Nisbett et al. (2012). *Intelligence: New findings and theoretical developments.* American Psychologist.
- UNICEF (2019). *The State of the World's Children 2019: Children, Food and Nutrition.*
- World Health Organization (2023). *Micronutrient deficiencies: Iodine and brain development.*

Further Reading for Parents & Educators

- Frederick Douglass. *Narrative of the Life of Frederick Douglass, an American Slave.*
- George Washington Carver. *How to Grow the Peanut and 105 Ways of Preparing It for Human Consumption.*
- Trisha Gura (2010). *Nutrients and Intelligence: The Micronutrient Connection.* Scientific American.

ABOUT THE AUTHOR

Catrina (Gooden) Ravenel—widely known as **Mineral Momma**—is a retired military veteran trained at the U.S. Air Force School of Aerospace Medicine in Ohio, where she completed comprehensive public-health training for Air Force personnel.

She earned her bachelor's degree in social work from Georgia State University and has dedicated her life to serving families as a literacy advocate and global health activist.

Her mission became deeply personal when her son was born with a severe learning disability. Refusing to accept the limitations placed on him, she searched tirelessly for natural, science-supported ways to strengthen his mind and elevate his IQ.

His transformation revealed her calling: to help millions of families reclaim their children's potential and restore generational health and longevity through natural healing solutions that work.

She is the founder of **Minerallymade LLC**, a movement rooted in the transformative truth that we are made of minerals—not disease.

Through Minerallymade, Catrina empowers parents to rebuild their children's brilliance and at the same time heal entire families by replenishing what deficiencies have stolen and break the cycles of imbalance that lead to dysfunction.

Catrina's message is both urgent, hopeful and powerful:

You are not diseased-made—you are Minerallymade.

I appreciate you too!

2:15

Weekly Search Insights Newsletter

09.06.2025 - 15.06.2025

Subscribed

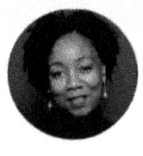

Stolen Intellect
askmineralmomma

Views	Followers	Likes
1.35M	**29.7K**	**115K**
+25.1K	+482	+1.72K

One of your posts outperformed **99.5%** of other creators in search results!

BONUS CHAPTER

STOLEN INTELLECT, RECOVERING THE MISSING LINK TO GENERATIONAL HEALTH

All my research was paying off. Once I discovered the missing link to my son's learning disability was a simple nutritional deficiency, and in just a few short weeks, my son's IQ significantly soared. Do other parents know they can easily increase their children's IQ and improve their comprehension, speech, reading, math and understanding I wondered.

There are millions of children who struggle with regular education too. You know them because they struggle in the classroom, with comprehension, speech impediments, but have no medical diagnoses, but struggle just the same. Our children are not slow or dysfunctional. But for these children to reach their highest human potential, their young brain needs minerals early in life or as soon as possible.

Mother Nature holds all the minerals and resources we need for eternity. Although Mother Nature is everywhere, we have eyes but strangely do not see her! Why? Because powerful institutions indoctrinated and manipulated us to be dependent on them for knowledge, understanding and information as if they were Divine Intelligence.

Tragically, Mother Nature was cut off to us and so was her infinite wisdom and intelligence. Like a thief in the night, our knowledge and intellect of Mother Nature was hidden and stolen in plain sight. "Who stole our knowledge of Mother Nature?" Sadly, we do not even think about asking because we didn't know we were robbed in the first place!

Family, I wrote this book to share with you my unique perspective about nature and its connection to our intelligence, good health, and longevity in that order. As you begin reading, start by imagining yourself holding the world in the palm of your hands or as if you're looking down into a globe.

From this perspective you now have the advantage of looking down into your hands and down into the world. Look closely until you see the players in the earth's game of life. The players are the people vs. deception.

The scenario is Isaiah 60:2 – where darkness covered the earth and gross darkness (ignorance) covered the people. Deception's weapon: Manipulation (He who controls the information, controls the world)! The People's weapon: Accessing the power of Divine Intelligence so together we can build a genius nation, increase generational good health, so we can increase our longevity.

How do people recover after their minds were hijacked, their health compromised, and their knowledge stolen? Collectively, the people must continue to activate their divine power and Divine Intelligence so they can fight to their strength but first they must know what their strength is.

We have a serious family problem. A lack of knowledge problem.

Knowledge is POWER and the solution is simple. Yes, a solution.

STOLEN INTELLECT I - BOOK REVIEW

This book has everything I've waited for all my life. Truths hidden in plain sight, healing remedies that no one will teach you, and a deep dive into knowledge that feels like reclaiming a stolen birthright.

Stolen intellect by Catrina Ravenel is not just a book - it's a powerful awakening. Ravenel doesn't merely skim the surface of natural wellness; she plunges into the heart of what your body truly needs to heal and thrive.

From the often-overlooked benefits of iodine and selenium to the critical importance of detoxing and nourishing the body at a cellular level, this book arms you with knowledge that has been kept from us for far too long.

Review by Martha M. Bello

A SPECIAL THANKS TO MY READERS

From the heart of **Mineral Momma** to every reader who turned these pages: thank you.

You could have chosen distraction, but instead you chose truth. You could have clung to labels, but instead you dared to look deeper. You chose to open this book, wrestle with hard realities, and believe that healing and intelligence are your birthright. For that, I honor you.

This book was not written for shelves or statistics. It was written for *you*—for the mothers who want their children to rise, for the fathers who refuse to accept brokenness as normal, for the families ready to reclaim what was stolen.

Without your eyes, your hope, and your courage, these words would remain ink on a page. You have breathed life into them.

Remember: you are **Minerallymade.** You were created with brilliance in your bones and wisdom encoded in your cells.

You are not a disorder or disease—you are the firmament, minerals, light, and potential. My prayer is that every lesson you carry from these chapters becomes nourishment for your home, fuel for your mind, and strength for your generations.

Thank you for walking this journey with me. Thank you for believing that health and genius belong to us, too.

May your children shine with clarity, and may you never forget—you are not diseased-made, you are **Minerallymade.**

With a perfect love,
© *Trina aka Mineral Momma*

WE ARE MINERALLYMADE- NOT DISEASED MADE

Above all systems of man exists an ancient Cosmic Recipe—
governing our biology, shielding our lineage, and determining
the strength passed from one generation to the next.

We were crafted from the earth,
nourished by the sea,
strengthened by the sun,
and sustained by the breath of life.
Across nations, cultures, and languages,
the human body speaks the same truth.

We are minerallymade! One Biology. Many Tongues.

English
We are Minerallymade.
Spanish
Estamos hechos de minerales.
Chinese
我们是矿养匠造的
French
Nous sommes façonnés par les minéraux.
Portuguese
Somos feitos de minerais.
Italian
Siamo fatti di minerali.
German
Wir sind aus Mineralien gemacht.

Arabic
نحن مكوّنون من المعادن.
Hindi
हम खनिजों से बने हैं।
Japanese
私雕刁叮烦贰方房递督爹颠跌抵犊大
Korean
우리는 미네랄로 이루어져 있다.
Russian
Мы созданы из минералов.
Greek
Είμαστε φτιαγμένοι από ορυκτά.
Yoruba
A jẹ́ ohun tí ilẹ̀ àti òkun dá.
Wolof
Ñu ngi joge ci suuf ak ndox.

We are Minerallymade — not disease-made.

Enjoy these convenient links to order your supplements or reference material mentioned in this book.

Red Palm Oil | Organic reviews
Sale Price $11.99

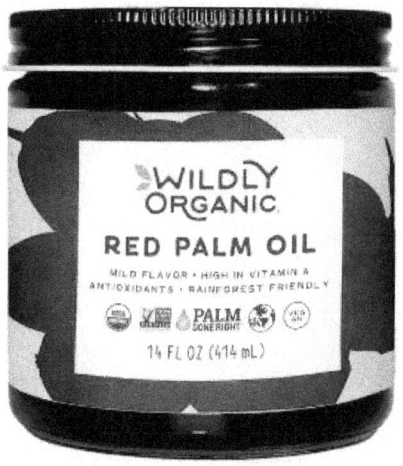

Buy 1 to use as a lotion
Buy 1 for the kitchen
Link
https://i.refs.cc/kxYSekHs?smile_ref=eyJzbWlsZV9zb3VyY2UiOiJzbWlsZV91aSIsInNtaWxlX21lZGl1bSI6IiIsInNtaWxlX2NhbXBhaWduIjoicmVmZXJyYWxfcHJvZ3JhbSIsInNtaWxlX2N1c3RvbWVyX2lkIjozMzYwODMwODJ9

Cod Liver Oil

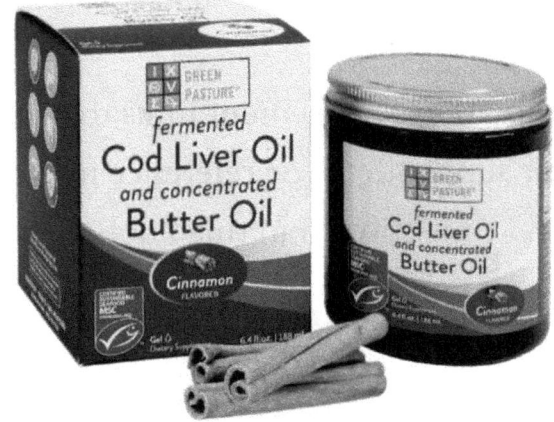

Link
https://amzn.to/3HRDwjW

Wakame Cut Seaweed 2.5 ounce

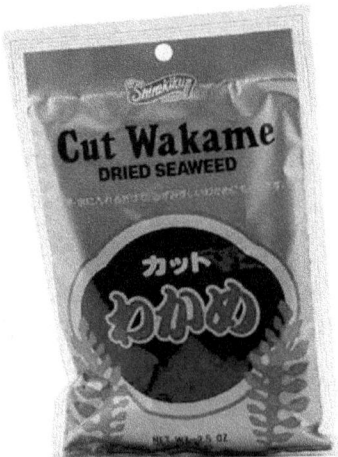

Link to buy
https://amzn.to/4ggaG9s

Wakame Recipe:

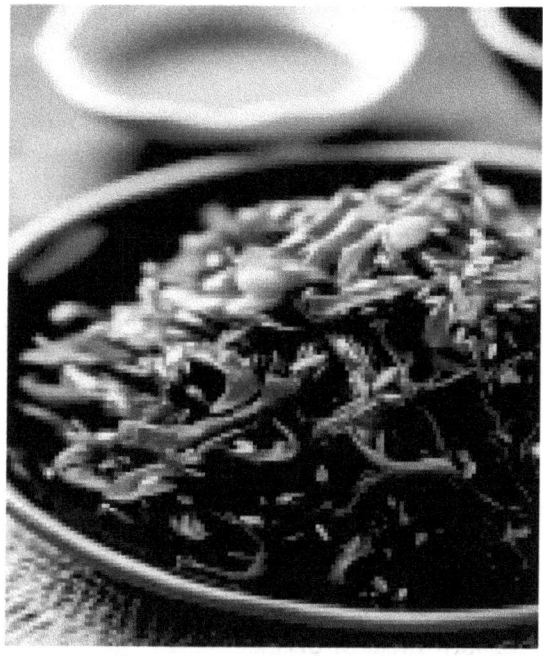

To reconstitute: Place ½ cup seaweed in warm water for 10 minutes; Squeeze some lemon juice (citric acid) in water. (citric acid reduces the arsenic that is naturally occurring is seaweed but not good for human health). Drain and rinse once more. **Wakame** expands two to three times its dry volume and turns a brighter shade of green.

I personally, like to add about ½ cup onion.
Lightly sprinkle across the top nutritional yeast, turmeric, and cayenne pepper to taste. Drizzle toasted sesame seed across the top then stir. Whole sesame seeds are optional. Keep refrigerated.

I make enough for the week so each day, I add 2 tablespoons of wakame to soups, or I eat about ¾ cup wakame salad with a meal or by itself.

Remember a little seaweed goes a long way. It's time we make seaweed as a part of our meals.

MIYEOK GUK – A KOREAN TRADITION

Seaweed Soup for Postpartum Mothers

New mothers in Korea have a large bowl of seaweed soup up to three times a day for 1 month. Seaweed cleanses blood, detoxifies the body, helps the womb contract and increases breast milk. A staple postpartum soup recipe packed with nutrient rich ingredients that aid in healing and hydration for mom and nourishes the baby's brilliance.

Ingredients

- 1.5 ounces dried miyeok (wakame) yields about 3 cups soaked
- 6 ounces beef stew meat or brisket
- 2 teaspoons minced garlic
- 2 tablespoons soup soy sauce (gukganjang, 국간장) If unavailable, use 1 T regular soy sauce and season with salt to taste
- 1 tablespoon sesame oil
- salt and pepper
- 10 cups of water

Instructions

- Soak the dried miyeok (wakame) per package instructions (usually 10 to 20 min) or until miyeok turns soft and plump. Rinse twice. Drain well and cut into bite sizes.
- Cut the beef, seafood, or tofu into thin bite size pieces. Marinate with 1 tablespoon of soup soy sauce, garlic, and a pinch of pepper.
- Heat a large pot over medium high heat. Sauté the meat with the sesame oil just until the meat is no longer red.
- Add the miyeok and 1 tablespoon of soup soy sauce and continue to sauté for 4 to 5 minutes.

- Add 10 cups of water and bring it to a boil. Skim off any scum. Add salt and pepper to taste. Lower the heat to medium low. Boil, covered, for 20 to 30 minutes until the meat is tender and the broth is slightly milky.

Traditional Korean Postpartum | Ancient Recipes & Practices

MORE LINKS

Beet Powder	Link	https://amzn.to/3HWRqB2
Boron	Link	https://amzn.to/47iyhnD
Cod liver Oil/Adults	Link	https://amzn.to/47UdvuE
Cod Liver Oil/Kids & Adults	Link	https://amzn.to/47UdvuE
Dulse	Link	https://amzn.to/3Vsm4W8
Grapeseed oil	Link	https://amzn.to/4n71eHD
Iodine/Ioderol 12.5	Link	https://amzn.to/3UUka0s
Iodine/J. Crows Lugols	Link	https://amzn.to/3HBAMXN
Kelp (kombu)	Link	https://amzn.to/4g7Jeea
Magnesium	Link	https://amzn.to/4ntnE6n
Mozuku	Link	https://amzn.to/46ohSwS
Mushroom Agaricus Blazei	Link	https://amzn.to/4g8ZfjI
Ozone Water Machine	Link	https://amzn.to/3UWFS3P
Salt - Baja Gold	Link	https://amzn.to/4nbXWD3
Salt - Celtic	Link	https://amzn.to/4aqG9EX
Salt - TaTa (Iodized Salt)	Link	https://amzn.to/4nP9CMk
Selenium	Link	https://amzn.to/3JDIj8Z
Sulfur (MSM)	Link	https://amzn.to/3JGnOsn
Vitamin C	Link	https://amzn.to/46fHSdN
Wakame	Link	https://amzn.to/4nfgiDn
Zinc / oysterzinc *My favorite Zinc* (Selenium, copper, iodine & Zinc)	Link	http://www.marinehealthfoods.com/ discount code: **mineralmomma10** and receive 10% discount.

Book purchase: Stolen Intellect (recovering the missing link to generational health)	Link	https://amzn.to/4p2gmYF
Book: Dr. Afrika – African holistic health	Link	https://amzn.to/3I0j7co
Book: Dr. Brownstein *Iodine why you need it, why you can't live without it.*	Link	https://amzn.to/4g98dO2
Book: *The Iodine Crisis*: Lynne Farrow	Link	https://amzn.to/41FZbSG
Book: Selenium by Dr. Gerhard Schrauzer	Link	https://amzn.to/3V7IsnF
B1/B6/B12	Link	https://amzn.to/4ntnE6n
B2/3	Link	https://amzn.to/41zeKM2

Disclaimer: I have partnered with Amazon, and using these links is how I make a few cents on each purchase. These supplements and brands are the supplements I personally use and strongly advocate.

Thank you.

REVIEW TIME!

Congratulations!

You finished the book ☺

I look forward to reading your book reviews!

Please take the time to share your thoughts in the review section of Amazon, Goodreads, or google, or wherever you purchased the book, just don't forget to **leave a review!**

Potential customers love reading your reviews too. ☺

Health Coaching Service

I am here for you.

BRING THE MESSAGE TO YOUR COMMUNITY

If your organization is ready to awaken minds, nourish families, and restore generational health, I am available for:

- **National & International Conferences**
- **Women's Empowerment + Maternal Health Events**
- **Men's Wellness & Leadership Gatherings**
- **K–12 Schools & Literacy Programs**
- **Colleges, Universities & Public-Health Departments**
- **Churches, Ministries & Community Faith Events**

Book me to speak, teach, ignite, and elevate. Let's restore intelligence, family, and future — one community at a time.

SPEAKING & TEACHING ENGAGEMENTS

Available for:

- Conferences
- Women's Events
- Men's Events
- Schools & Educational Programs
- Colleges & Universities
- Churches & Faith-Based Gatherings

Healing testimonials
Send to:
www.weareminerallymade.com

FOLLOW ME

YOUTUBE
@AskMineralMomma

Stolen Intellect

https://www.youtube.com/@AskMineralMomma

Instagram
@ask_mineral_momma

TikTok https://www.tiktok.com/@askmineralmomma?_t=ZP-8zjQ146ELL4&_r=1

I appreciate you!
DONATIONS ARE WELCOMED
Please send to:
Cashapp $Mineralmomma222
Or
ZELLE: CATRINARAVENEL@YAHOO.COM

Contact Information:

weareminerallymade.com
catrinaravenel@yahoo.com
minerallymade@gmail.com

INDEX

SECTION I

A

ADHD (attention deficit hyperactivity disorder), **62, 73, 86**

Africa, iodized salt strategies, **33, 39–40, 76–77**

Alps, iodine deficiency in (1788), **25–26**

American literacy crisis, **31–32, 72–73, 75**

Autism spectrum disorder, **62, 86**

B

Behavioral disorders, nutritional origins of, **31–32, 72–75**

Birth defects, iodine deficiency and, **35–36, 61–63**

Brain development
— prenatal, **35–38, 53–55, 60–62**
— postnatal, **36–38, 85–87**

Breastfeeding, iodine and toxin transfer through, **35–36, 62–63, 66–67**

C

Cadmium exposure, **62–63, 66–68**

Cancer, iodine and selenium protection, **36–39, 63**

Central Asia, iodized salt education (Kazakhstan), **29–31, 78–79**

China, universal salt iodization, **40–42, 78**

Choline, prenatal brain development, **61–63**

Cod liver oil
— historical public health use, **36–38, 82–87**
— pregnancy benefits, **65–66**

Congenital iodine deficiency, **25–27, 46–47**

Cretinism (iodine deficiency disorder), **25–26, 30–31, 56, 99**

D

Developmental delays, nutritional causes, **31–32, 46–48, 61–62**
Disability, preventable intellectual, **25–27, 30–31, 56–57**

E

Education failure, biological roots of, **31–32, 34–36, 72–75**
Ethiopia, iodized salt law (2011), **39–40, 76–77**

F

Fat-soluble vitamins (A, D, E, K), **36–38, 57, 85–87**
Fertility decline, iodine deficiency and, **35–36, 46, 61**
First 1,000 days, brain vulnerability during, **60–62**

G

Generational intelligence, mineral foundations of, **26–27, 34–36, 56–58**
Gestational diabetes, iodine deficiency and, **64–65**
Goiter
— endemic, **25–26, 30, 47–49**
— Great Lakes region, **44–49**
Great Lakes (U.S.), iodine-depleted soils, **44–46**

H

Heavy metals (lead, mercury, cadmium), **62–63, 66–68**
Hyperthyroidism (iodine repletion concerns), **59**

I

Illiteracy, biological causes of, **31–32, 72–75**
Infant mortality, iodine deficiency and, **35–36, 61**
Intellectual disability, preventable, **25–27, 30–31, 56–57**
Iodine
— discovery (1811), **25**
— deficiency, **25–27, 30–32, 44–49**
— pregnancy requirements, **35–36, 60–62**
— thyroid function, **35–37, 53–55**
Iodine Global Network (IGN), **33, 39, 78**
Iodized salt
— history, **25–26**

— global programs, **29–32, 39–42, 76–79**
— U.S. policy failure (1948), **51–52, 59**

K
Kazakhstan, school-based iodine literacy, **29–31, 78**

L
Language delay, iodine deficiency and, **31–32, 46–48, 61–62**
Learning disabilities, nutritional origins, **25–27, 31–32, 46–48**

M
Maternal nutrition, iodine and intelligence, **35–36, 60–62**
Memory formation, iodine and selenium, **35–37, 53–55**
Miscarriage, iodine deficiency and, **35–36, 46, 61**

N
Neurodevelopment, mineral regulation of, **35–38, 53–55**
Neurons
— dendrites, **53–55**
— synapses, **53–55**

P
Pica, mineral deficiency signal, **73–74**
Placenta, toxin transfer across, **62–63**
Policy failure, U.S. iodine protection, **51–52, 59**
Prenatal vitamins, iodine absence in, **61–62**

R
Reparations, public health (concept), **111–113**

S
Salt iodization
— effectiveness, **29–32, 39–42**
— economics of prevention, **58–59**
Selenium, thyroid and brain protection, **35–37, 53–55, 63**
Speech delay, iodine deficiency and, **31–32, 46–48**
Switzerland, iodine transformation, **25–27**

T

Thyroid hormone (T3, T4), brain development role, **35–37, 53–55**
Toxic exposure, prenatal, **62–63, 66–68**

U

UNICEF, iodized salt campaigns, **29–31, 39–40, 78–79**
United States
— Goiter Belt, **44–49**
— iodized salt introduction (1924), **49–50**
— policy reversal (1948), **51–52**

W

Women's health, iodine deficiency and, **35–36, 46–47, 61–65**
Womb, first site of intelligence formation, **35–36, 53–55, 60–62**

SECTION II & TESTIMONIALS

A

Assembly Bill 418 (California Food Safety Act), **122**
Accountability, institutional absence of, **123–124**
Acetylcholine (learning and memory), **173**
Aggression, malnourished brain and, **125–126**
AIDS/HIV, selenium support in, **161–162**
Air pollution, prenatal neurodevelopmental impact, **200**
Alzheimer's disease, **169, 173–174**
Antioxidants
— selenium-dependent enzymes, **158–167**
— vitamin E as cellular shield, **140–157**
Aspartame
— pregnancy exposure concerns, **126**
— cancer associations, **126–127, 129**
— "Zero" labeling warning, **126–127**
Astigmatism (personal testimony), **136**

B

Behavior, malnutrition-linked changes, **125–126**
Blindness, preventable, **134–137**

— vitamin A deficiency, **134–136**
— red palm oil restoration, **135–136, 143**
Blood vessels, vitamin C and capillary strength, **147–149**
Boswellia (frankincense), **173–174, 177–178**
— memory and inflammation support, **173–174**
Breast health
— iodine storage in tissue, **202–203**
— prevention vs detection, **208**
Bromate (potassium bromate), **122–125**
Brownstein, David, M.D.
— iodine therapy and thyroid health, **201–207**
— breast tissue iodine sufficiency, **202–203**
— iodine–selenium safety framework, **158–167**
— alignment with cancer recovery testimony, **197–199**
Brain
— malnourishment effects, **125–126**
— adult cognitive decline, **169–170**

C

Cancer
— potassium bromate carcinogenicity, **124–125**
— prevention vs awareness critique, **132–133**
— selenium and iodine protective framework, **158–170**
— **testimony: recovery following iodine and selenium supplementation, 197–199**
Cardiomyopathy
— selenium deficiency (Keshan disease), **160–161**
Celebration culture (awareness vs prevention), **130–133**
Chemical additives, industrial food system, **123**
Children
— vision loss risk, **135–137**
— behavioral outcomes linked to nutrition, **125–126**
Cod liver oil
— cognition and ancestral prevention testimonies, **180–183, 194–195**
Crime scene metaphor (America), **123**

D

Dialysis statistics, **123**
Disabilities awareness critique, **132–133**
Divine Intelligence framework, **127, 132–133, 194–195**
Doctors and institutions, critique of, **130–133, 185–187**

E

Eczema and skin healing (red palm oil), **140, 150**
Erectile dysfunction
— testimony and circulation protocol, **211–212**
Eggs (ovarian), formed in utero, **195–197**
Endocrine disruptors, **123, 200**

F

Fat-soluble vitamins (A, D, E), **140–157**
Fireworks pollution (heavy metals), **197, 200**
Fertility
— iodine and menstrual regulation, **204–205**
— testimonies of restoration, **204–205**

G

Genocide framing (systemic poisoning language), **122–123**
Glutathione peroxidase (selenium enzyme), **166–167**
Goiter prevention (iodine–selenium balance), **169–170**

H

Hearing loss prevention, **143–145**
Heart disease
— selenium protection, **160–162**
— fluid-inflammation model, **151**

I

Iodine
— removal from flour, **122**
— breast tissue protection, **202–203**
— thyroid regulation, **201–207**
— topical first aid use, **191–193**

— **cancer recovery testimony (with selenium), 197–199**
Immune system resilience, **150–152, 161–162**
Institutions, synchronized failure of, **185–187**

K
Keshan disease, **160–161**
Kidney disease disparities, **123**

L
Lugol's iodine (J. Crow's), **191–193, 206, 211**
Lymphedema, selenium therapy, **159–160**

M
Magnesium
— menstrual pain relief, **205**
— glutathione support, **204**
Malnourished brains, **125–126**
Mastectomy critique, **202–203**
Memory
— sage and Boswellia support, **173–174**
Millet
— metabolic and cardiovascular support, **174–179, 212–214**
Mothers' Wit (ancestral healing testimonies), **194–200**
MSM (with vitamin C), **148–149, 205, 211**

N
Night blindness, **135–136, 143**
Nosebleeds (vitamin C deficiency), **145–150**
Neurodegenerative disease risk, **169**

O
Off-gassing (new car chemical exposure), **199, 212–213**
Oxidative stress, **150–152, 169**
Ozone water (circulation claim), **211**

P

Palm oil
— red palm oil (vitamins A & E), **135–157**
— oxidized vs fresh, **154–156**
Patient vs victim terminology, **122**
Perchlorate exposure, **197, 199–200, 206**
Potassium bromate
— global bans, **122**
— U.S. allowances, **122**
— toxicity evidence, **124–125**
Pregnancy
— nutrient depletion, **195–197**
— iodine and selenium protection, **201–207**
Prevention vs detection, **132–133, 208**
Prostate health
— testimony and restoration protocol, **211–214**

R

Rat experiment (nutrition deprivation), **125–126**
Red palm oil
— vision, skin, nerve repair, **135–140, 150–157**
— personal testimony, **138**
Remission critique, **137, 203**

S

Sage (Salvia officinalis), **173–174**
Schrauzer, Gerhard N., Ph.D.
— selenium and cancer prevention research, **158–167**
— glutathione peroxidase and antioxidant defense, **166–167**
— cardiomyopathy (Keshan disease), **160–161**
— immune system and viral disease research, **161–162**
Selenium
— cancer protection framework, **158–167**
— immune and viral defense, **161–162**
— pregnancy and placenta, **162**
— **cancer recovery testimony (with iodine), 197–199**
Seizures (oxidative stress model), **150–151**

Soil mineral depletion, **158, 167**
Strokes and recovery support, **158–161, 174**

T
Testimonies
— **cancer recovery (iodine and selenium), 197–199**
— cod liver oil and cognition, **180–183**
— menstrual cycle restoration (kelp and minerals), **204–205**
— erectile dysfunction recovery, **211–212**
Thyroid
— iodine dependency, **201–207**
— selenium conversion (T4→T3), **161**
Tocopherols vs tocotrienols, **152–154**
Toxic exposures (industrial food, air, water), **123**

V
Vitamin A
— blindness prevention, **134–137**
— hearing protection, **143–145**
Vitamin C
— nosebleeds and capillary integrity, **145–150**
— iron absorption, **147**
Vitamin E
— retina and brain protection, **140–157**
Vision loss, **134–142**

W
Women's health
— mineral depletion, **187–188**
— breast and womb protection, **201–210**

www.ingramcontent.com/pod-product-compliance
Lightning Source LLC
Chambersburg PA
CBHW080517030426
42337CB00023B/4552